A PHOTOGRAPHIC
·GUIDE TO·
CONFORMATION

A PHOTOGRAPHIC
·GUIDE TO·
CONFORMATION

ROBERT OLIVER
AND BOB LANGRISH

J. A. ALLEN

First published in Great Britain by
J. A. Allen & Co. Ltd
1 Lower Grosvenor Place
London SW1W 0EL

Reprinted 1991
Reprinted 1992
Reprinted 1993

British Library Cataloguing in Publication Data
Oliver, Robert *1940–*
    A photographic guide to conformation.
    1. Livestock: Horses
    I. Title II. Langrish, Bob
    636.1

    ISBN 0–85131–522–4

Designed by Paul Saunders
Layout by Alan Hamp
Line drawings by Dianne Breeze

Typeset by Phoenix Photosetting, Chatham
Printed and bound in Great Britain by
Butler & Tanner Ltd, Frome and London

CONTENTS

To my brother
the late Leonard William Oliver

Acknowledgements

I would like to thank the following people for their kindness and help with this book:

my wife Ali:

the Biddlecombe and Wellon families;

Giles Hine;

Lesley Gowers, for her expertise and patience in the preparation of the text for the publishers, J. A. Allen;

and last but not least, Bob Langrish for his patience whilst photographing the numerous subjects which appear in this book.

Robert Oliver

Publisher's acknowledgements

The publishers are grateful to Peter Goody for allowing them to use his excellent book, *Horse Anatomy*, as a source of reference for the illustrations; and to Dianne Breeze for supplying the line drawings.

INTRODUCTION

An eye for a horse

In years gone by dealers and old stud grooms were the best judges of a horse. Nowadays the only way to acquire an eye for conformation is to study as many different horses as possible. It helps to spend time at horse shows and sales looking at exhibits, ideally with someone experienced beside you. Reading as many books as possible can be useful too, as can visits to local riding stables where all types and sizes are available. In fact, all equestrian activities offer the keen young judge the opportunity to gain experience, and only by asking questions and discovering the answers will you really learn. Those who ride have the added advantage of being able to compare ride with conformation. Always remember that you can improve a horse's way of going but you cannot alter its basic conformation.

Recognising a young unfurnished animal's potential is often extremely difficult, especially if you are not told of its breeding. If a correctly made horse in poor condition is fed and worked correctly, over a period of time he will fill out properly, whereas a wrongly made horse, regardless of condition, cannot be put right.

Fat or gross condition can hide a multitude of faults. Points to look for in a thin horse are: good movement; withers that are higher than the top of the quarters; reasonable width of chest; short back; good straight hind legs; and a tail set on well even though the quarters may not be well developed. When viewed from the side, the horse should appear to have plenty of front although the show-jumping fraternity prefer a shorter front. Often horses in poor condition still show quality and presence.

Conformation in relation to performance

Correct conformation is important to the horse not only in work but also at rest. Horses stand on their legs for a great proportion of their lives; they also rest standing up as well as lying down. A well-put-together horse will be naturally balanced both ridden and loose, with movement that reflects his physique. His performance should far exceed that of a badly made horse. Moreover, he should enjoy a longer working life because he is mechanically more efficient. Conformation does, of course, vary according to the purpose for which the horse is required – speed, stamina or weight-carrying capacity – but whatever his chosen sphere a horse with a combination of good points should find it easier to work and stay sound. Nevertheless one cannot entirely ignore a horse because of his looks – there have been countless odd-shaped individuals who have more than proved the point that 'Handsome is as handsome does'.

Disagreement between experts

People will always disagree about the finer points of horses. However, whilst no two judges will have quite the same idea about perfection, on the weak points of a horse no good judges should differ.

The racing industry always favours good forelegs and shoulders together with straight action, as this combination leads to fewer training problems. On the other hand, the hunting fraternity are keen on depth of girth and good, clean hind legs, as riding in deep going, jumping in awkward places and carrying a rider all day can mean that the hind leg is the first area to suffer injury.

Disagreements often arise over the weight-carrying capacity of a horse. It is bone below the knee not height that carries weight. But most will agree that up to 8 inches of bone will carry 13 stones, that 8–9 inches will carry between 13 and 15 stones, and that a real heavyweight horse up to any weight should have over 9 inches of bone. All judges will agree that quality of bone is desirable. Flat, flint-like bone with well-defined sinews is preferable to round, soft, common bone. When measuring bone, take a tape and measure round the top of the cannon bone, just below the knee.

The pastern, into which the fetlock runs, acts as a shock absorber. If it is short and upright, it will be less efficient in this respect. If unduly long, the ride will be soft and comfortable but, eventually, if given an excess amount of work, will show weakness. Hunter people dislike long pasterns. This particularly applies to the hind joints. As they become enlarged the horse knocks them and the skin can get broken. With the wind and wet of winter, infection soon sets in, thereby producing a lame horse.

Splints, large and small, are always a matter of opinion, as are filled legs and capped hocks.

Sway- and dippy-backed horses are unsightly without a saddle and have weaknesses of the back. They are not usually the best of jumpers or hunters, but they invariably give a good ride. Ladies are more prone to forgive a dippy back than men. The odd show horse with such a back is either first or last depending on the judge.

OVERALL CONFORMATION

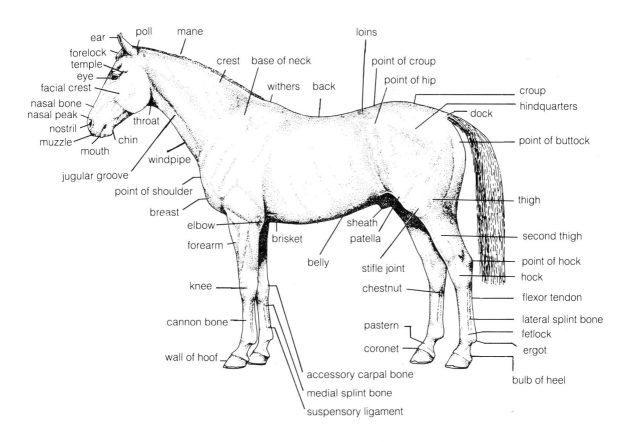

Points of the horse.

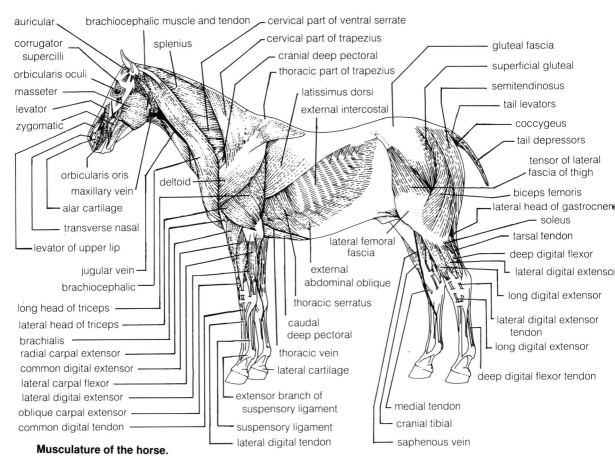

auricular
corrugator supercilli
orbicularis oculi
masseter
levator
zygomatic

brachiocephalic muscle and tendon
splenius

cervical part of ventral serrate
cervical part of trapezius
cranial deep pectoral
thoracic part of trapezius
latissimus dorsi
external intercostal

gluteal fascia
superficial gluteal
semitendinosus
tail levators
coccygeus
tail depressors
tensor of lateral fascia of thigh
biceps femoris
lateral head of gastrocnemius
soleus
tarsal tendon
deep digital flexor
lateral digital extensor

orbicularis oris
maxillary vein
alar cartilage
transverse nasal
levator of upper lip

deltoid

jugular vein
brachiocephalic

long head of triceps
lateral head of triceps
brachialis
radial carpal extensor
common digital extensor
lateral carpal flexor
lateral digital extensor
oblique carpal extensor
common digital tendon

lateral femoral fascia
external abdominal oblique
thoracic serratus
caudal deep pectoral
thoracic vein
lateral cartilage

extensor branch of suspensory ligament
suspensory ligament
lateral digital tendon

long digital extensor
lateral digital extensor tendon
long digital extensor
deep digital flexor tendon

medial tendon
cranial tibial
saphenous vein

Musculature of the horse.

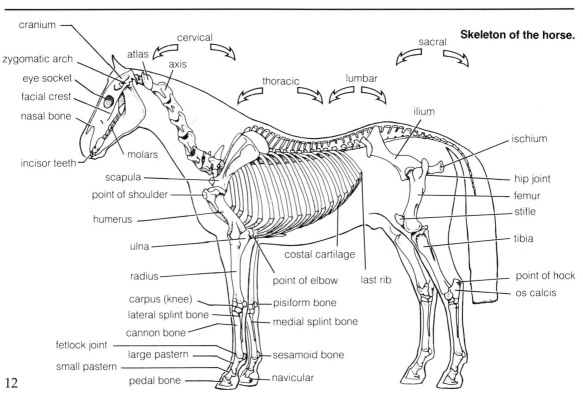

cranium
zygomatic arch
eye socket
facial crest
nasal bone

cervical
atlas
axis

sacral

Skeleton of the horse.

thoracic
lumbar

ilium
ischium
hip joint
femur
stifle
tibia
point of hock
os calcis

incisor teeth
molars
scapula
point of shoulder
humerus
ulna
radius
carpus (knee)
lateral splint bone
cannon bone
fetlock joint
large pastern
small pastern
pedal bone

costal cartilage
point of elbow
pisiform bone
medial splint bone
sesamoid bone
navicular

last rib

12

A quality thoroughbred horse which, although lacking condition and muscle, is basically correct. With proper work and feeding this horse would develop well. One to buy in the rough.

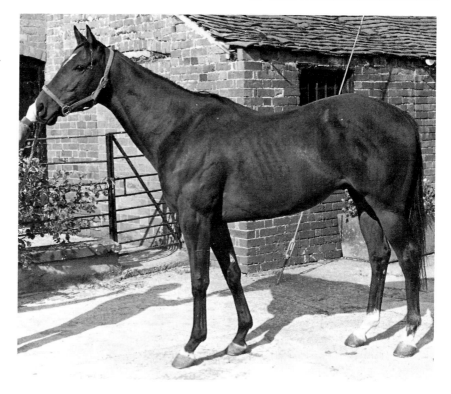

A thoroughbred horse whose conformation is less than desirable. His head and neck are 'upside down'; his shoulder is straight; he has a roach back and a very poor-shaped hind leg. No amount of condition could disguise these faults.

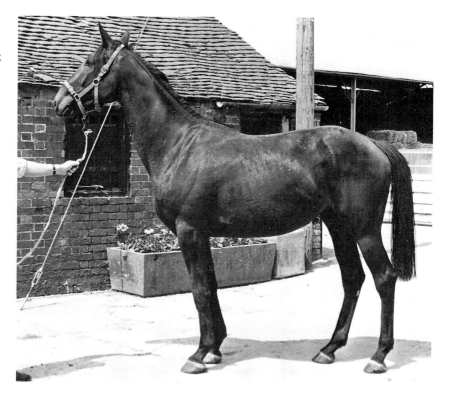

A plain, common-bred horse. The pasterns are short and upright; the foreleg is back at the knee; the croup is high and goose-rumped; the horse is very narrow above the hocks, lacking second thigh. Although this animal has plenty of faults his head and neck are passable for his type.

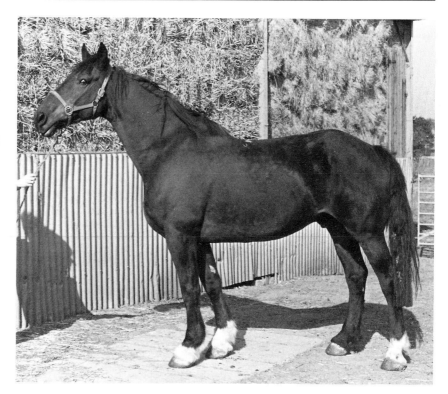

BELOW: An attractive, quality horse in superb condition, and a big winner in the show ring. He has an excellent set of limbs, clean and free from any blemishes. He has a good front, a well-set-on head and neck, is deep-bodied with well-sprung ribs. Ideally the tail could be set on a little higher. He has four good feet in proportion to his overall size.

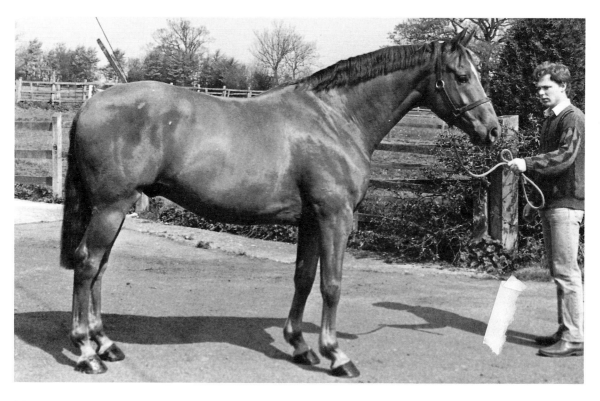

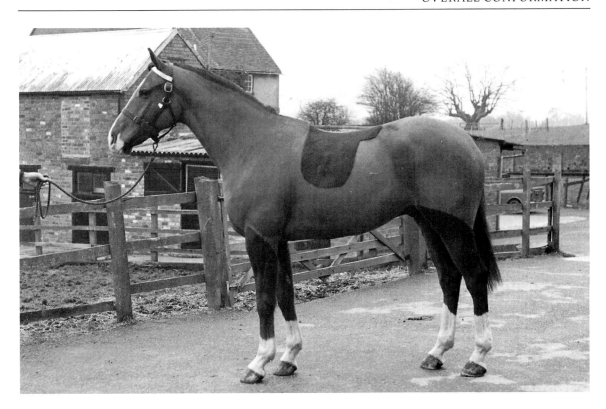

ABOVE: Everything right. A champion ridden hunter and champion working hunter, sold to Switzerland to show jump. A horse that is correctly put together with everything in proportion. Pictured the day after a hard day's hunting. A well-muscled, fit horse.

RIGHT: Everything wrong. A horse in show condition, with no room for further improvement. He appears bosomy, and his forelegs are placed too far underneath him, emphasising the fact that he is back at the knee. He has long cannon bones, straight pasterns and is straight-shouldered. He is inclined to be sway-backed and his hocks are too far behind him. To compensate, he has a lovely head and neck and a lot of people would like to own him.

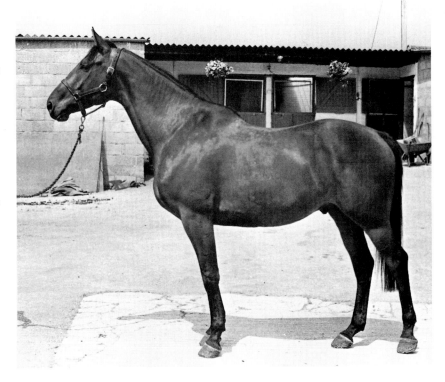

A cobby type with a short neck and a straight shoulder.

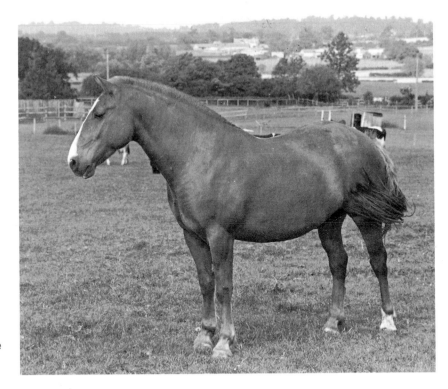

BELOW: A common type, standing 15.1 hh. Notice the straight foreleg and the hooking hind leg.

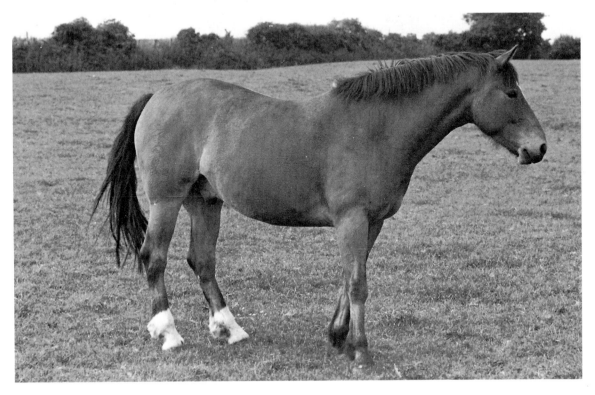

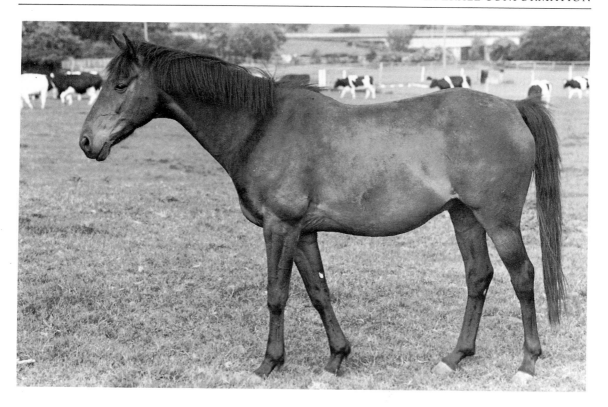

ABOVE: Another common type. This individual has a straight shoulder, is light of bone below the knee and has no second thigh.

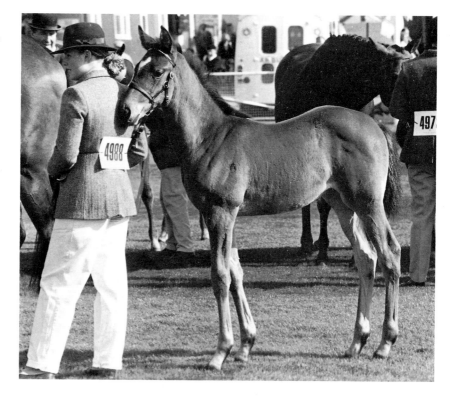

A hunter foal just a few months old. He has correct limbs and a nice slope to his shoulder. His back is short and he has a good outlook.

A hunter yearling in good condition. He has clean limbs, a good length of front and a nice outlook.

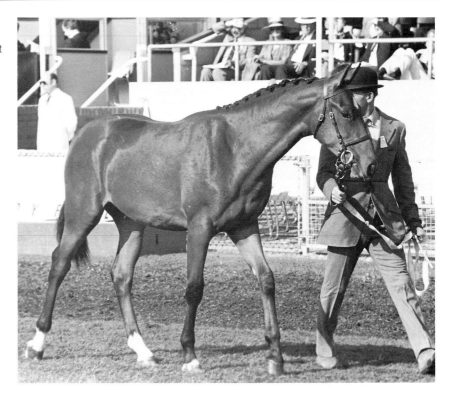

BELOW: A twenty-two-year-old pony. Note the dipped back and the long curly coat, usually attributed to age. The pony is correctly made and in his younger days would have been an attractive animal.

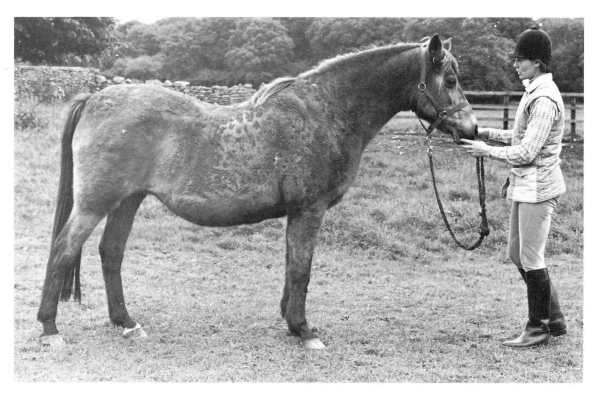

THE BODY

The body should be deep through the heart, making the animal appear short-legged. A good animal grows larger to the eye as you get closer to him. Horses which are light and narrow through the middle are described as 'showing daylight', especially if 'on the leg'. They will run up light and stand little work. Short backs have strength and weight-carrying capacity, while the opposite can be true of long backs.

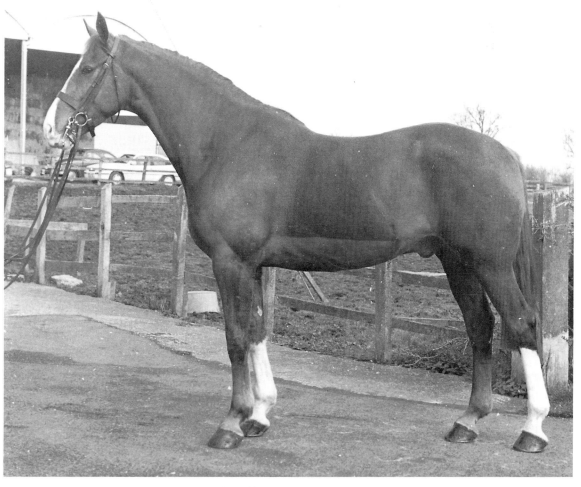

A well-proportioned horse with a good short back and nice depth.

A well-proportioned champion pony mare with depth, scope and compactness.

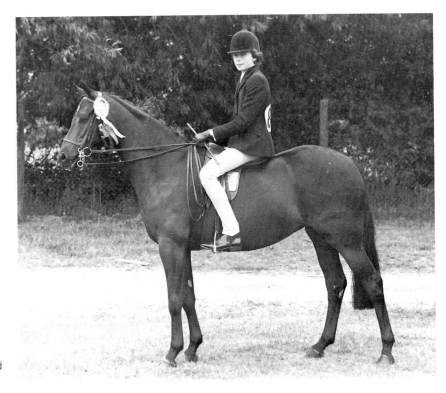

BELOW: This horse is long in the back (note the length behind the saddle). It would be 'on the leg' when fit.

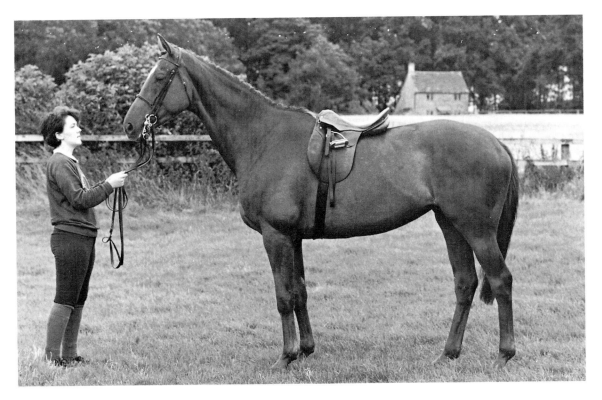

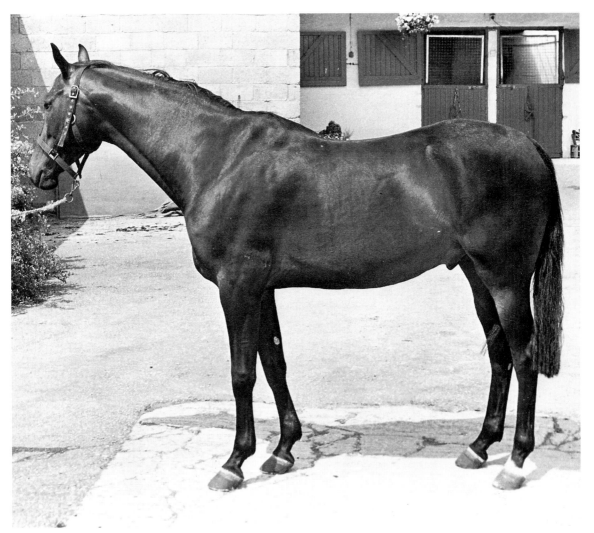

This horse is shallow through the girth (some would say tubular, especially if in light condition). The animal is in show condition, but no amount of condition will increase the depth through the girth.

THE BACK

The back, or middle part of the horse's anatomy, is defined as between the withers and the hip. It should be short and compact for strength, and there should be plenty of depth through the heart. The short-coupled horse is the one which will not only carry weight, but still also hold condition. The long-backed horse is invariably weak and will probably be slack over the loins as well. However, most mares are usually slightly longer in the back than geldings and stallions.

In outline the back should be almost level. Occasionally roach-backed (the opposite of hollow-backed) horses are seen. Rarely do they make good competition horses as they can be difficult to saddle and uncomfortable to ride.

A quality thoroughbred horse showing a nice, short back with plenty of depth and well-sprung ribs.

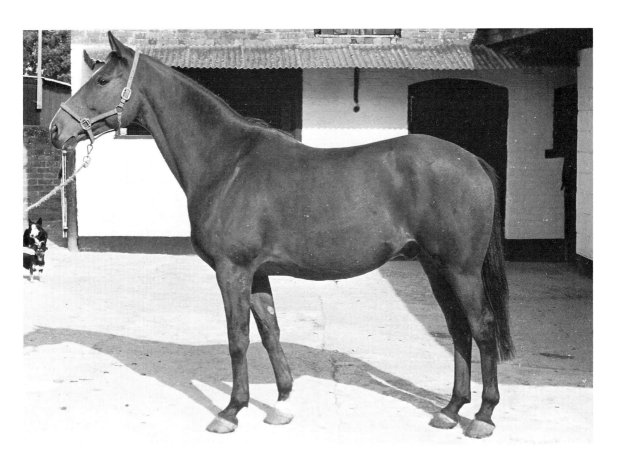

A hunter type, again showing a short back with plenty of depth, together with strong loins. This horse carried 18 stone two days a week throughout the hunting season.

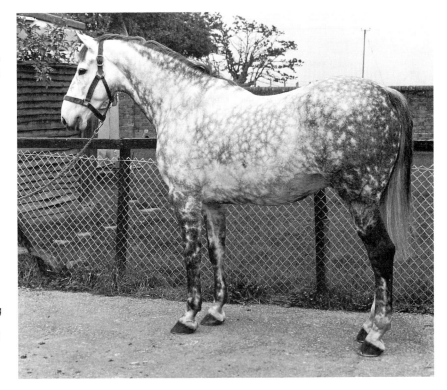

BELOW: A long-backed, weak-loined animal, tending to be herring-gutted. This type would run up very light after a day's hunting. A tendency also to be flat-sided.

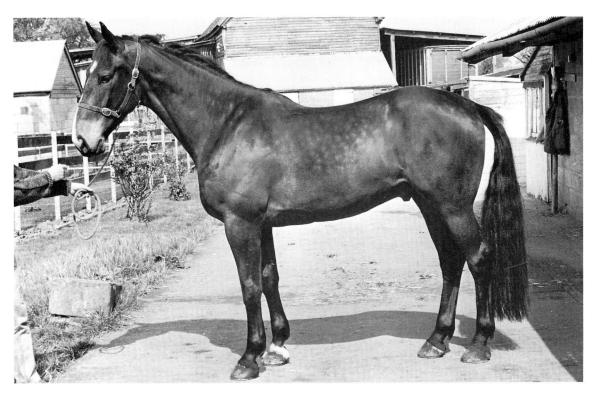

This horse's back is short but also rather tubular and hollow. It also has a loaded shoulder.

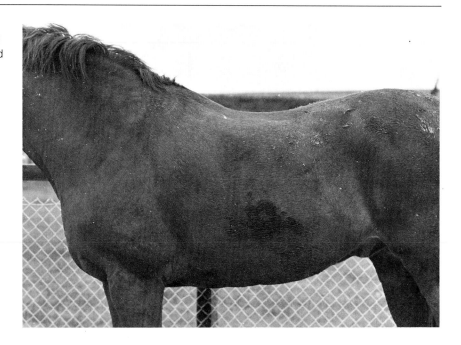

A back that is hollow or dippy makes for a comfortable ride but it is a bad fault and a weakness. This picture shows a good example of a dippy back.

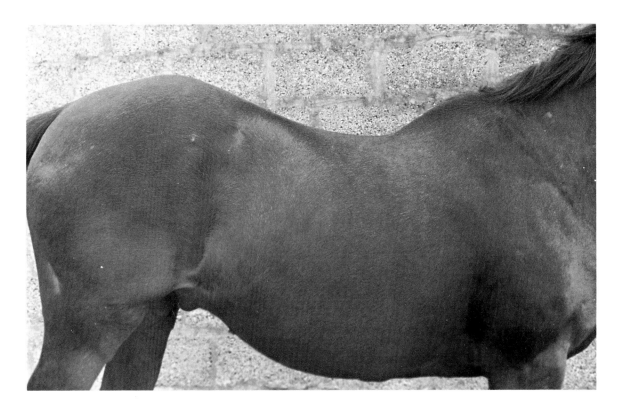

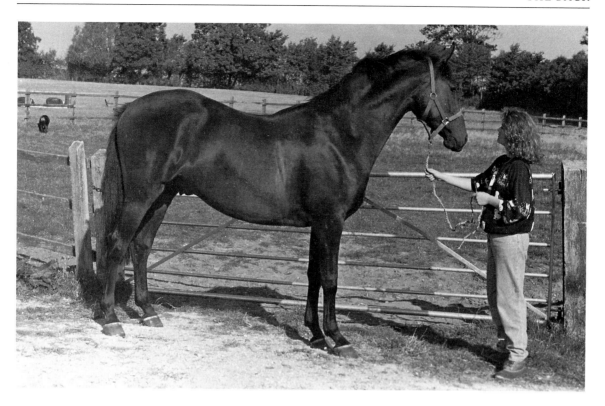

ABOVE: A young horse with a sway back; he is also lower in front. With age this horse's back could worsen.

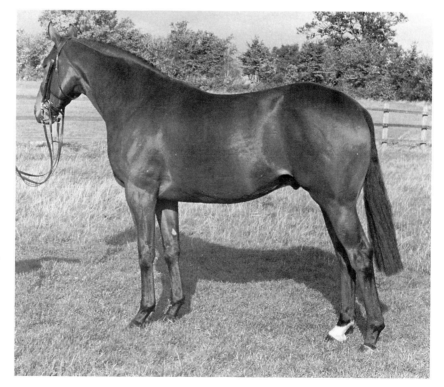

A good short back, well-sprung ribs, and nice hindquarters with length from the hip to his pin, and with good length from the hip to the hock. Altogether a well-proportioned horse and with the right amount of bone to carry his body. This horse was a champion young hunter in Britain and Ireland and was later sold to go show jumping. He stood 16.2 hh and had 8½ inches of bone below the knee.

HINDQUARTERS AND TAIL CARRIAGE

The hindquarters should be strong, well-developed and muscular. There should be generous length from the hip to the hock, together with good, strong, muscular second thighs, always an indication of power and strength, since the hind end is the propelling force.

A well-set-on tail, carried well away from the hocks, is essential for the looks and balance of the horse. Animals which have a low tail carriage and sloping quarters are unattractive. In former days, dealers would resort to underhand methods to make horses carry their tails higher.

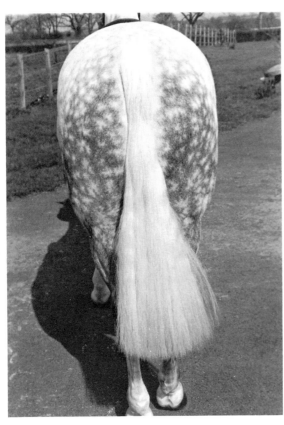

Good, level hips; lovely round hindquarters; exceptional second thigh and well-set-on tail. An old-fashioned groom might describe this back end as 'pear-shaped'.

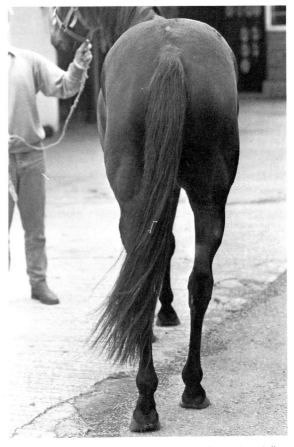

Narrow hindquarters, sloping away to a low-set-on tail.

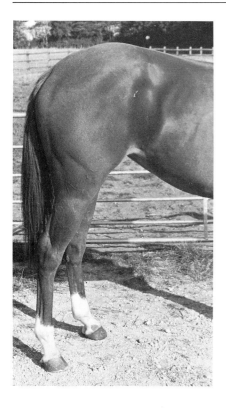

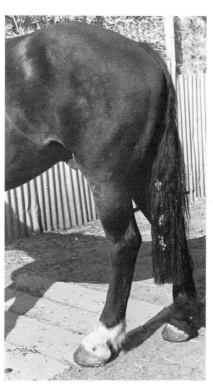

FAR LEFT: Weak quarters and loins.

LEFT: A 'jumper's bump' on a common horse. Note also the poverty line.

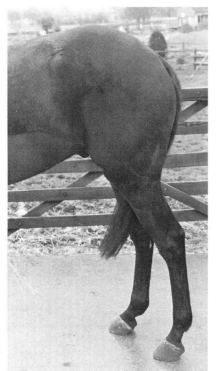

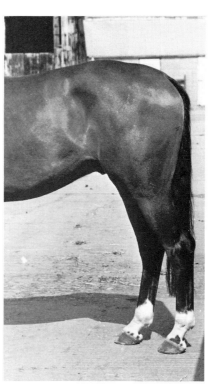

FAR LEFT: A high croup with a low-set-on tail.

LEFT: Flat hindquarters with no muscle and weak loins.

TAIL CARRIAGE

People do not generally like to see an exaggeratedly high tail carriage, or tails that are carried straight out or sideways. Many regard these features as a weakness or a sign of back trouble – Arabs being the exception. Sunken tails and docks are equally undesirable.

Tail swishing is an indication of resistance or discomfort, which is very undesirable in the show ring and penalised in the dressage arena.

Fine, thin docks indicate quality breeding, whereas short, thick, heavy docks indicate commonness. Viewed from behind, a well-carried tail should swing loosely from side to side with the movement of the horse.

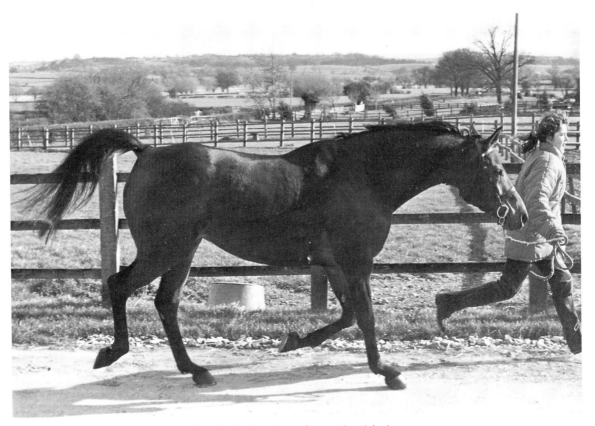

The high tail carriage of a part-bred Arab.

HIND LEGS AND HOCKS

Of all the points of conformation, many consider the hocks and hind leg to be the most important. Since the hind legs provide the power for the entire body, it is essential that the quarters are well let down into strong hocks and that the hocks should be as near to the ground as possible, with short cannon bones. There should be plenty of length from the hip to the hock. Viewed from the side they should not be excessively straight nor bent at too much of an angle, indicating weakness. An imaginary vertical line drawn from the point of the buttock to the ground should touch the hock and the back of the fetlock joint.

BELOW: Hind legs, viewed from the side. **(a)** Good hind leg, length from hip to point of buttock and from hip to hock; good gaskin (second thigh); clean well-let-down hocks. **(b)** Sickle hock, light of bone, no second thigh; cut in above hock. **(c)** Hocks up in the air; short from hip to point of buttock and from hip to point of hock; cut in above hock. **(d)** Overstraight hocks.

RIGHT: Hind legs, viewed from the rear. **(a)** Good. **(b)** Split up and poor – note poverty line; hocks up in the air. **(c)** Cow-hocked, no second thighs.

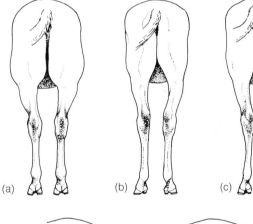

(a)　　　(b)　　　(c)

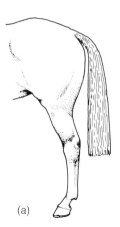

(a)

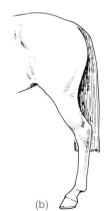

(b)

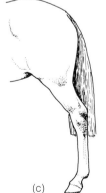

(c)

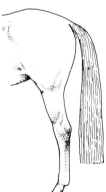

(d)

Two examples of good
clean hind limbs, with
length from hip to hock and
well-defined hocks and
pasterns.

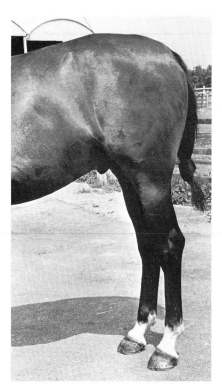

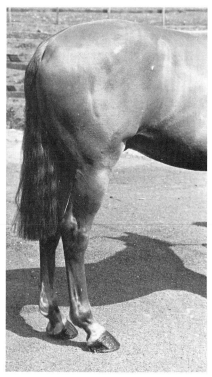

RIGHT: An overstraight hind
leg, which if subjected to
excessive concussions and
strain would be prone to
spavins.

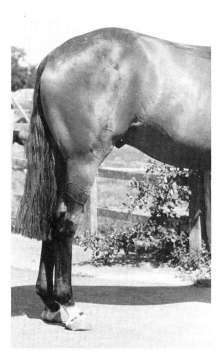

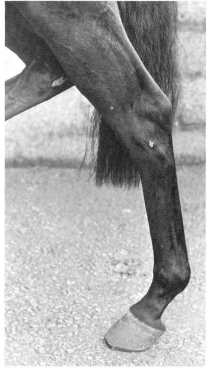

FAR RIGHT: A bent hock, with
long, weak, sloping
pasterns.

RIGHT: Round, thick, puffy hind joints. Also note the squared-off toes, which indicates that this animal drags its toes; and the enlarged bone spavin on the off hind. Bone spavins often occur in pairs and can cause acute lameness.

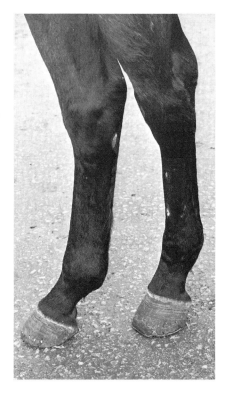

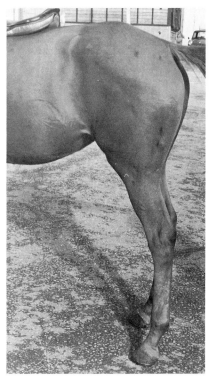

FAR RIGHT: This individual has weak hindquarters lacking in second thigh, long cannons and upright pasterns. Such small hocks could easily spring a curb.

RIGHT: A low-set-on tail, a jumper's bump and a bent hind leg.

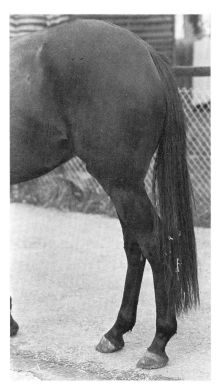

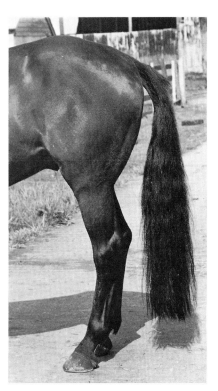

FAR RIGHT: A poor hind end which is goose-rumped and accompanied by sickle hocks. This horse's hocks were also very close together (cow-hocked).

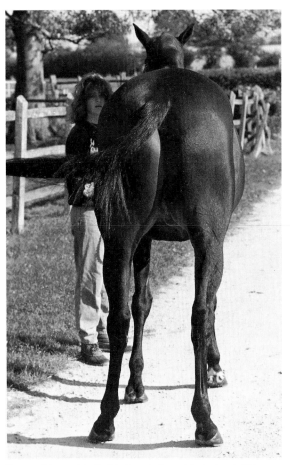

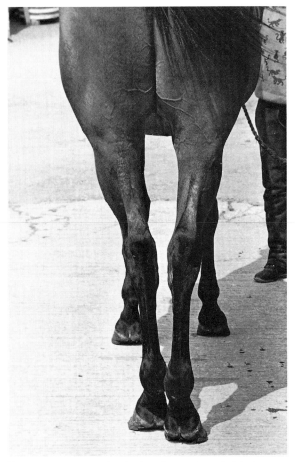

Base wide – wide behind and also wide in front. This individual is liable to give its rider a 'roly' sort of ride. Horsemen have often said of this sort: 'You could push a wheelbarrow between his limbs.' A lot of racehorses go wide behind when travelling at speed. Show ponies that over-move in trot sometimes go very wide behind to balance themselves.

Base narrow – cow-hocked and very close behind yet wide in front. In work, this horse could easily knock its fetlock joints and would probably always have to wear protective boots and be correctly shod by a knowledgeable farrier.

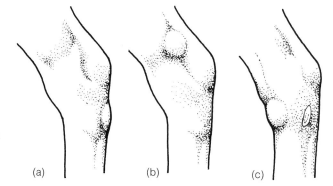

Unsoundnesses in the hock area. **(a)** Curb. **(b)** Thoroughpin. **(c)** Bone spavin.

(a) (b) (c)

HOCKS

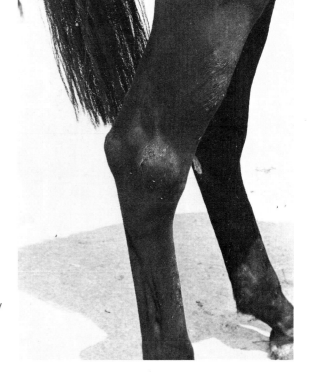

RIGHT: Bent hind leg with a thoroughpin. Thoroughpins are bursal enlargements which rarely cause lameness but are unsightly. Considered more of a blemish than an unsoundness, they extend right through the hock to the inside.

BELOW: Two examples of capped and puffy ill-defined hocks. A capped hock is not an unsoundness but is very unsightly. The enlargement can vary in size from an egg to a tennis ball. Caused mainly through insufficient bedding or through kicking the wall of the stable or horsebox whilst travelling.

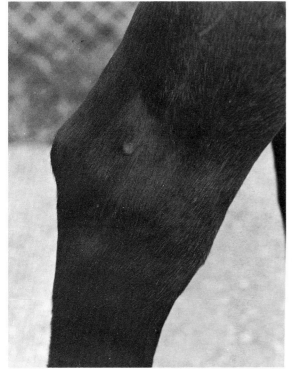

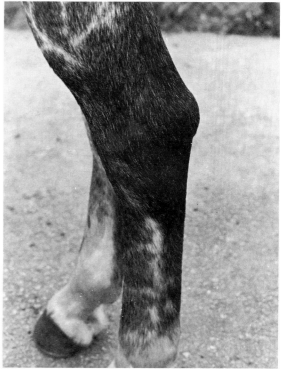

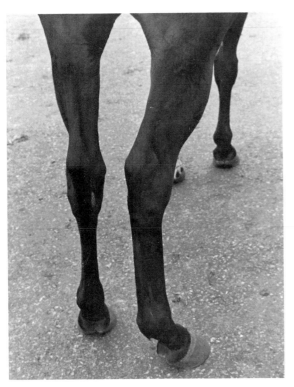

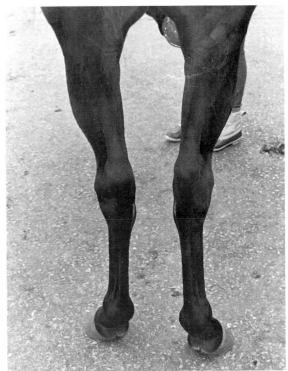

ABOVE: Two views of cow hocks taken from different angles. When viewed from behind, the hocks are very close together with the lower limbs turned out. Rarely do they interfere with the horse's performance in light work. They do not, however, indicate weight-carrying ability. Cow hocks are a weakness and unsightly. Note also this horse's puffy hind joints, calloused on the insides from brushing.

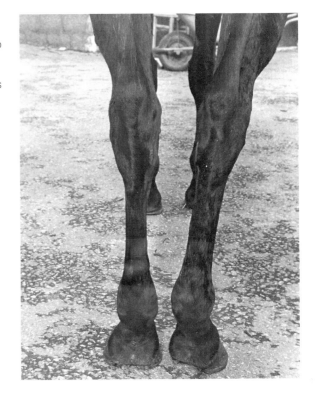

Hocks very close together. This horse's hind fetlocks show wear and puffiness.

CURBS

The presence of a curb can be seen about four inches below the point of the hock. Curbs can be either hereditary or 'man made' on a bad-shaped hock that is prone to this condition. Jumping awkward places out of deep going is often the cause. The phrase 'curby hocks' is frequently used to describe a sickle- or cow-hocked animal. Horses showing hock defects lack power of the hind limbs. Occasionally a curb can be seen on even the best shaped hock. Whilst large curbs are easy to spot, it is sometimes necessary to run a hand down the back of the leg to detect a smaller curb. Curbs are considered an unsoundness except by the racing fraternity, who accept them on the grounds that racehorses usually run on the forehand.

RIGHT: A clean hock with a curb that is easily seen.

FAR RIGHT: A smaller curb with a hock that shows wear.

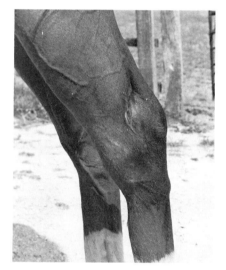
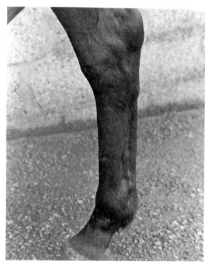

RIGHT: A long, fleshy, soft-looking curb. Its owner is very likely to go unsound.

FAR RIGHT: A bad, weak hind leg with a curby hock. 'Buyer beware'.

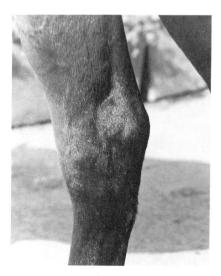
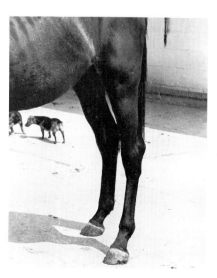

FORELEGS

A good muscular forearm is desirable. Viewed from the side it should be broad across the top. From the front to the point of the elbow, the forearm should taper gradually down to the knee. From the front it should be muscular on the outside and flat on the inside.

The knees should be large and flat. The cannon bone should be short, for strength, and broad and flat when looked at from the side. Below the knee the cannon bone and tendons should be of adequate width, in proportion to the size of the animal. The horse should neither be exaggeratedly over or back at the knee, the latter being the worse fault.

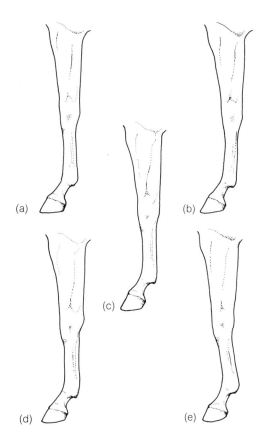

LEFT: Forelegs, viewed from the side. **(a)** Light of bone, long cannons, small knees, tied in below the knee. **(b)** Small knee, back at the knee. **(c)** Good foreleg, with good flat bone, large knees, fluted tendons, average pasterns, well-developed forearm. **(d)** Good foreleg. **(e)** Over at the knee.

BELOW: Forelegs, viewed from the front. **(a)** Good; short cannon bones. **(b)** Forelegs 'coming out of one hole'; turned-out feet; light of bone. **(c)** Bosomy and pigeon-toed.

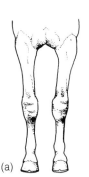 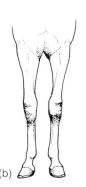 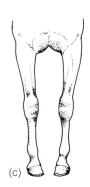

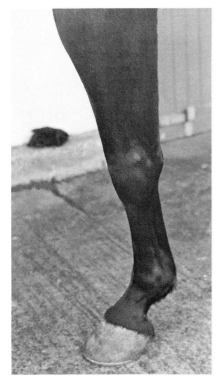 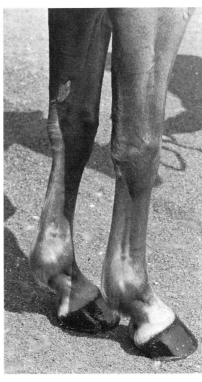

FAR LEFT: Good foreleg with muscular forearm. Ideally the foot could be one size larger.

LEFT: These forelegs are slightly long in the cannon bone. The foot is good and in proportion.

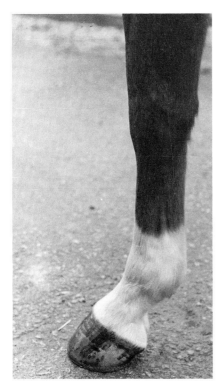 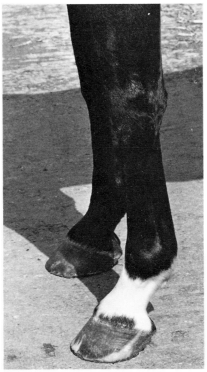

FAR LEFT: Excellent foreleg and very well-shod foot.

LEFT: Quality foreleg – excellent pastern, well-defined tendons and good flat bone. A little low in the heel.

RIGHT: Back at the knee. The whole foreleg appears concave. A very bad fault causing excessive wear to the back tendons. Very much disliked by knowledgeable horsemen in all competitive spheres.

FAR RIGHT: Over at the knee. This condition is preferable to being back at the knee as there is less strain on the tendons. However, if it is excessive it can be unsightly and is not favoured in the show ring. Many racehorses are slightly over at the knee, which trainers like as the legs can withstand more work.

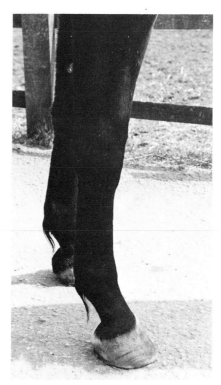

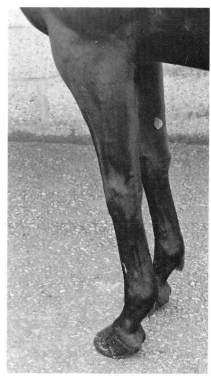

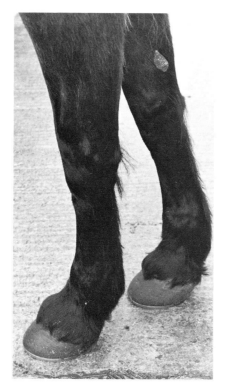

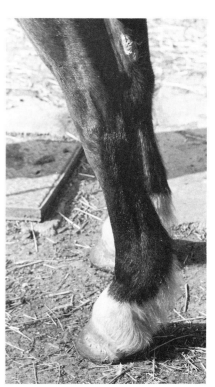

Two examples of common, coarse forelegs; back at the knee; short, upright pasterns; small round knees and joints.

RIGHT: A bad foreleg. A weak forearm running into long cannons, lacking bone below the knee. Very upright pasterns joining boxy feet. This horse would be described as light of bone.

FAR RIGHT: Round joints showing signs of ringbone on the pasterns. Note also the low, weak heels. This foreleg could be helped by regular shoeing, shortening of the toe and being shod longer at the heels.

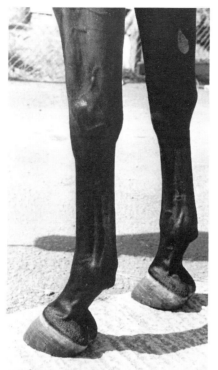

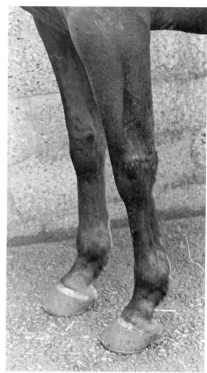

RIGHT: Bad tendon injury on an otherwise good foreleg.

FAR RIGHT: A horse with broken knees, due to a fall. He also turns his feet out, although he does not appear to be hitting his front joints as is usual in horses with this fault. A broken knee must be viewed with suspicion as a horse may be an habitual stumbler; on the other hand, the horse may have suffered an unavoidable accident.

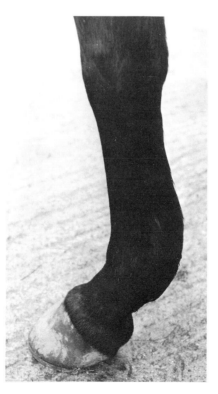

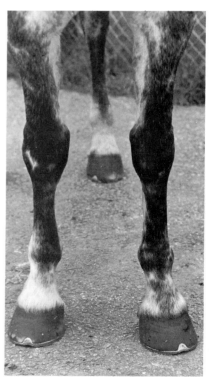

SPLINTS

Splints may be found on any part of the cannon bone. They occur more often in the fore than in the hind, and are more frequently seen on the inside than on the outside of the leg. Their position determines whether or not they will cause lameness.

A splint is a formation of bone thrown out as a result of overwork or injury from concussion. Splints will appear at any age in a horse's life though more usually in young, immature animals. Lungeing young horses on hard ground will undoubtedly add to the risk of splints.

The size of the splint can be from a tiny pin-head to an egg. Small splints, high under the knee, are often troublesome.

A splint well forward on the leg is considered far less harmful than one towards the back, where it might interfere with the tendons. Serious consideration should be given to large splints, since they may be bruised by the other foot and cause lameness.

Small splints are called 'peg splints'. Several splints together are called 'a chain'.

BELOW: Medium-sized splint close up to the knee.

BELOW RIGHT: Large splint on a horse that also turns its toes in. Horses with faulty action are the most liable to form splints, due to the extra strain.

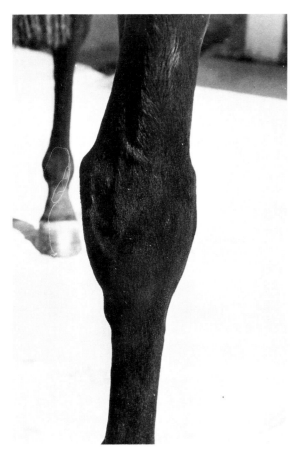

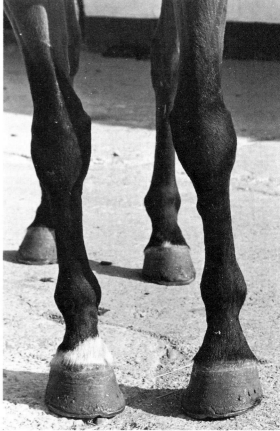

PASTERNS AND HEELS

The pasterns should be neither long nor too short and upright. If they are upright they act as poor shock-absorbers and often give an uncomfortable ride, especially on hard ground. Long, sloping pasterns give a comfortable ride but can have a tendency to show wear and puffiness. The ideal slope for a pastern is 45°.

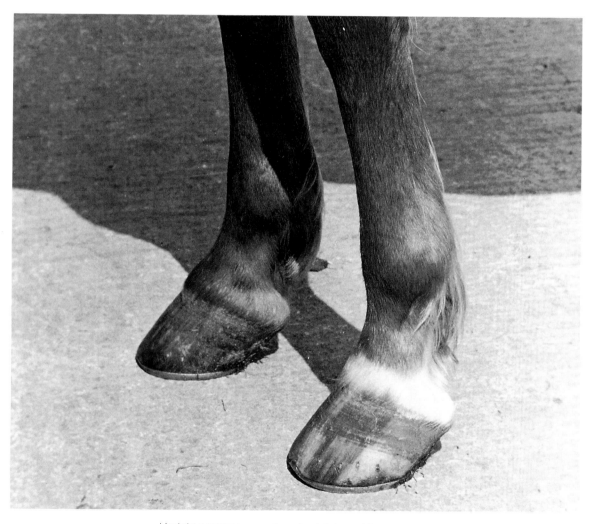

Upright pasterns, round appley joints and feet in need of shoeing.

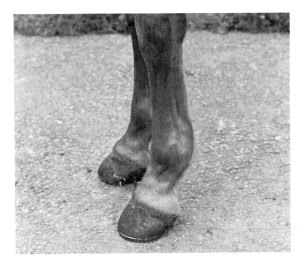

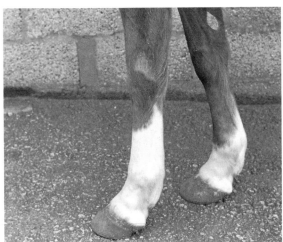

ABOVE: An upright foreleg, high of the heels.

ABOVE RIGHT: Low heels, upright pasterns and round joints – not good signs for wear.

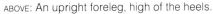

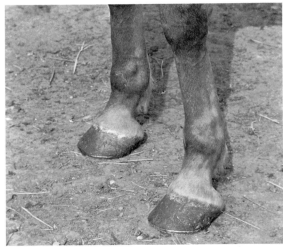

RIGHT: Upright pasterns, the legs showing signs of wear in the fleshy, puffy joints.

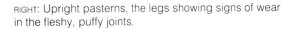

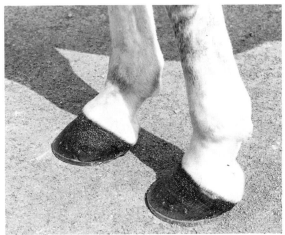

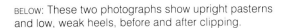

BELOW: These two photographs show upright pasterns and low, weak heels, before and after clipping.

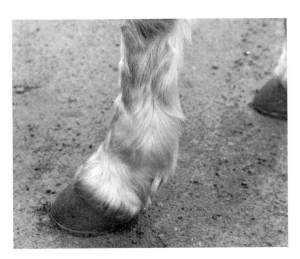

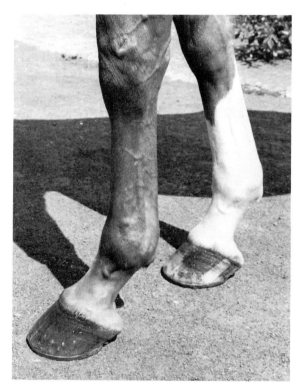

Long, sloping pasterns with a low weak heel. A long weak pastern will stand up to little work.

BELOW: Two pairs of forelegs with long cannon bones; they are therefore light of bone as well.

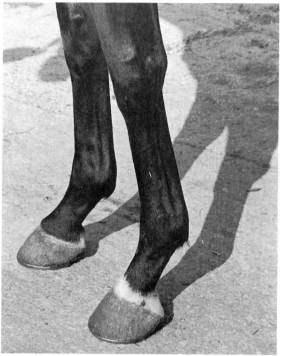

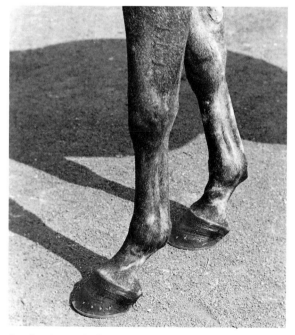

Another long, sloping pastern, belonging to a thoroughbred. Nice short cannon bones.

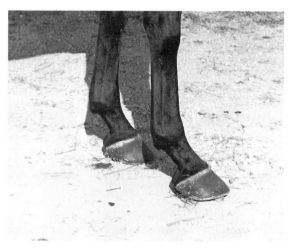

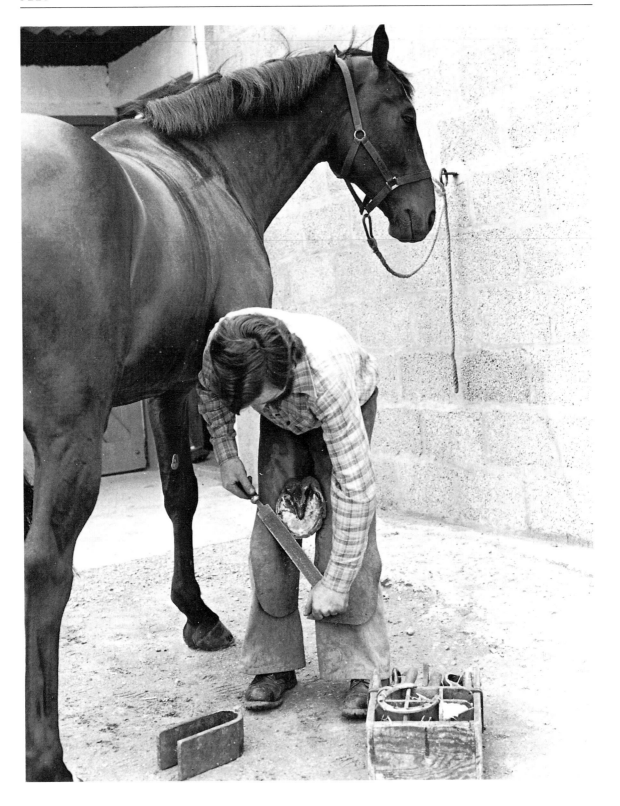

FEET

A horse should stand on four well-shaped feet which are in proportion to the size of the horse. The front feet should always be a pair; contracted or odd feet usually indicate trouble.

The frog should appear healthy and well developed. The frog acts as a shock-absorber as well as providing a foothold. It also has a role to play in assisting blood circulation.

Large, flat open feet often have heels that are too low. Animals with this type of feet could have difficulty crossing rough surfaces, as the soles of the feet can bruise easily; they are also prone to corns.

Low or dropped soles can come about as a result of laminitis. The feet of an animal suffering from, or having previously had, laminitis usually grow long at the toe and have rings on the wall of the hoof.

Small, boxy feet are frequently accompanied by contracted heels and are prone to navicular disease. Occasionally horses are born with small, upright feet which appear to be trouble-free. The hackney horse usually has small, upright feet.

Brittle, shelly feet are undesirable as they are difficult to keep shod correctly due to the breaking and splitting of the lower hoof. In some cases this is an inherited defect.

The shape of the foot is often determined by the conformation of the horse, but the old saying, 'No foot, no horse,' always holds true. It is unfortunate that many high-class horses suffer from foot trouble which renders them useless, whilst plain horses with good feet last longer.

To neglect feet is foolish and very much a false economy. Regular attention at all times, whether in or out of work, is important. A good farrier can work wonders by correctly dressing young horses' feet; he can also improve straightness in movement and the overall shape of the foot.

OPPOSITE: A good farrier is essential.

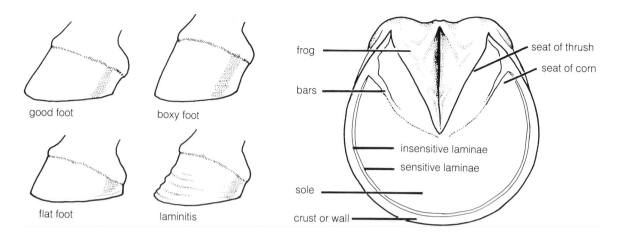

frog

seat of thrush

bars

seat of corn

insensitive laminae

sensitive laminae

sole

crust or wall

good foot

boxy foot

flat foot

laminitis

Feet.

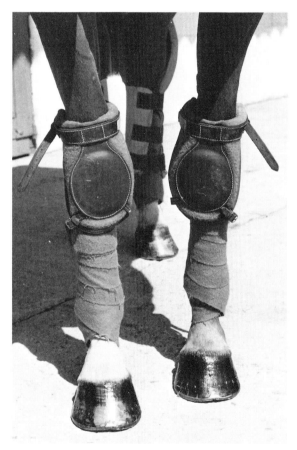

Excellent pair of front feet, nicely proportioned and well shod.

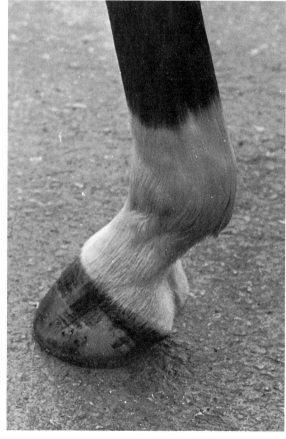

A well-proportioned foot on a very good foreleg. Note, however, that the toe may have been over-shortened, which is not a bad shoeing fault.

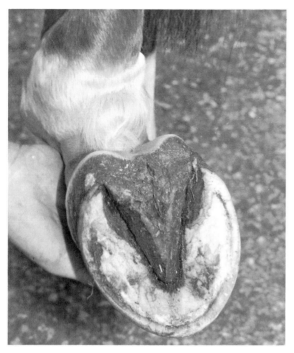

A well-developed sound frog on a strong, hard sole (hind foot).

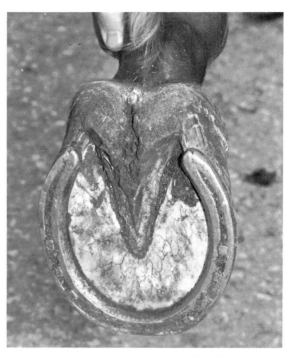

A frog which is not in the best of condition. The shoe could be slightly longer in the heel. Sound sole.

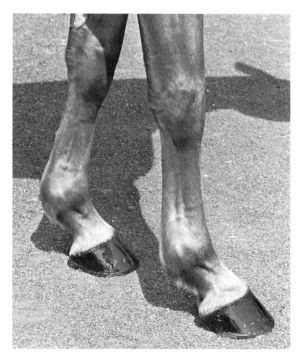

A good foot. Ideally the heel could be slightly higher and the toe shortened.

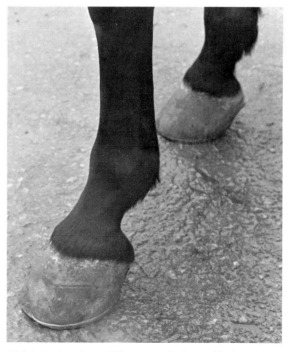

A high heel and smallish, narrow foot on a big horse.

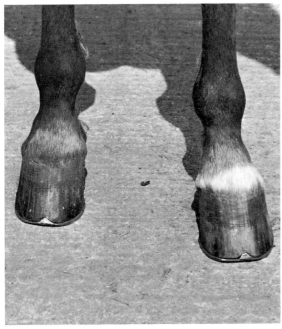

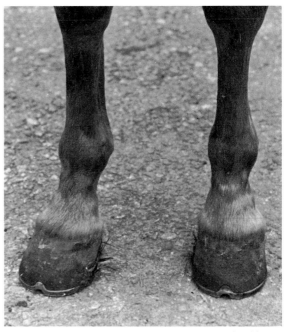

Small upright feet in need of shoeing. Suspect ringbone on the pasterns. Horses with short, upright pasterns are more prone to ringbone than those with sloping pasterns.

Upright feet; off-fore turns out, which could make this animal liable to brush. Well shod.

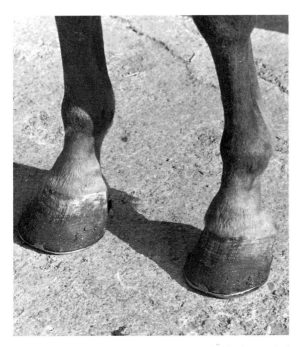

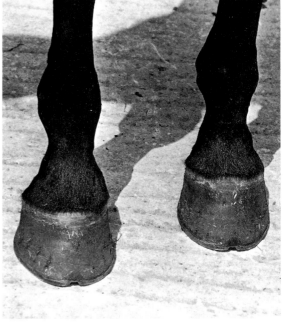

Flat-footed and inclined to turn inwards. Badly in need of shoeing.

Inclined to be concave; strong in the pasterns. Would recommend x-rays to discover true picture. Also note odd feet.

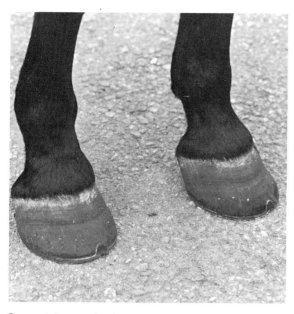

Suspect rings on hoof, and long toes in need of expert attention. This horse could have suffered from laminitis.

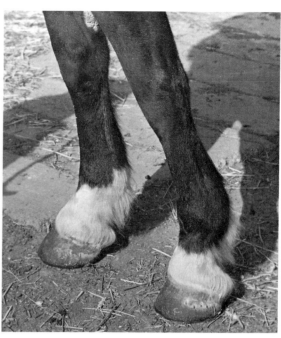

Small feet in relation to the limbs.

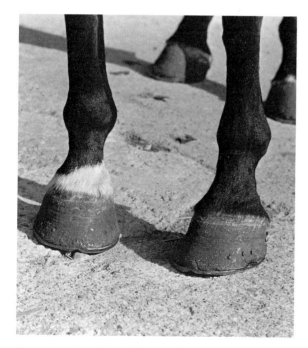

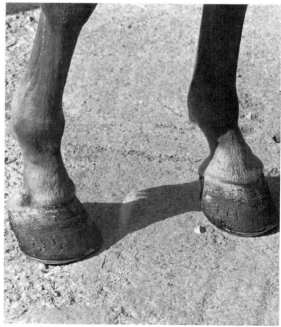

Two examples of turned-in toes. Twisted feet can be hereditary or due to neglect on the part of the owner. In young horses especially, every effort should be made to encourage the foot to assume the normal shape with regular attention from a good farrier.

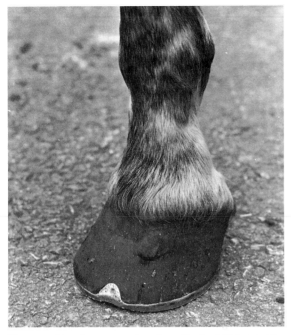

Damaged hoof, now growing down the foot. This could create a problem when in line for nailing. Note also the thickness on the pasterns.

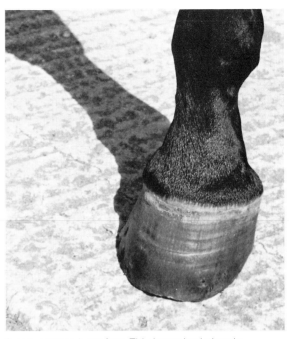

Small, narrow, boxy foot. This horse had chronic navicular.

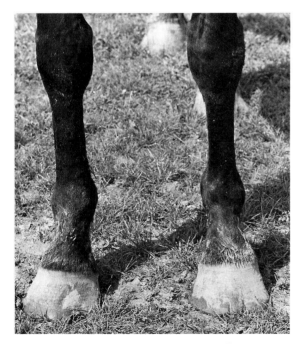

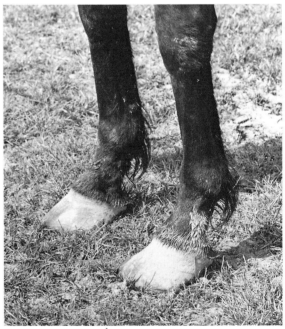

Two views of flat feet with low, weak heels. This horse's feet have been badly neglected while out at grass and are in urgent need of a farrier. Even at grass, horses' feet need regular attention, every six weeks.

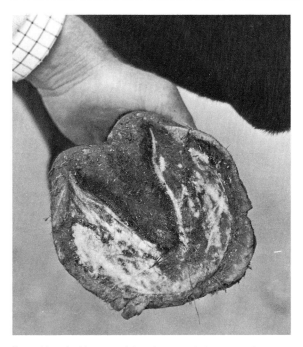

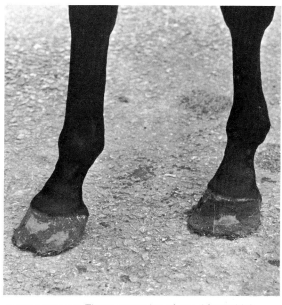

ABOVE AND BELOW: Three examples of good feet which have been badly neglected.

Sound hoof with a good frog but sorely in need of attention.

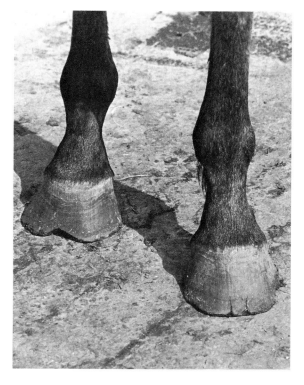

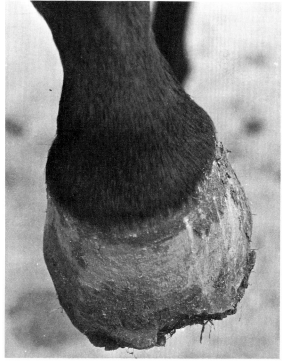

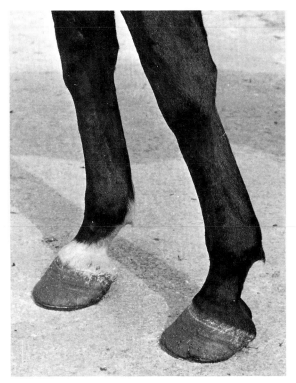

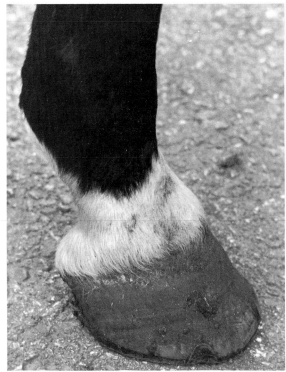

ABOVE: Low, weak heels and rings on the hoof wall. Correct shoeing could improve these feet.

ABOVE, RIGHT: This hind foot has been allowed to become over-long at the toe, which could cause an overreach. Note that this horse is prone to drag its toes.

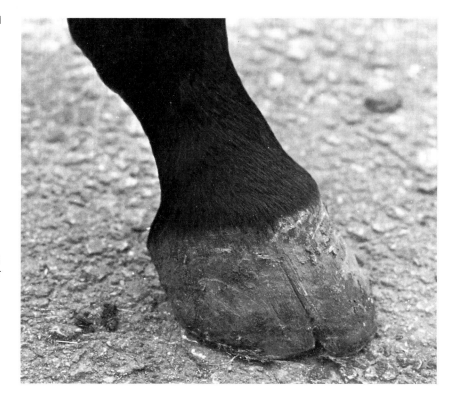

Hind foot with a nasty sand crack due to neglect. Other causes are improper distribution of weight caused by treading on uneven surfaces and turning horses out on wet ground. If grit is allowed to enter the crack, severe lameness will occur.

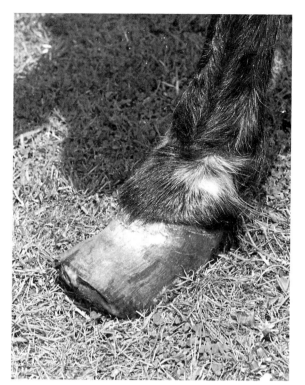

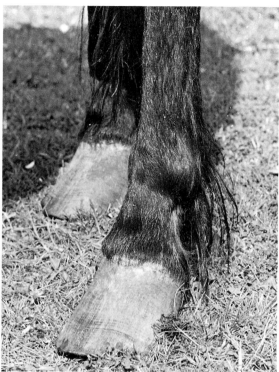

Fore foot of a horse with chronic laminitis.

The hind feet of the same animal, showing the altered angle caused by laminitis. Note the distortion and the rings of the hoof wall.

CHEST AND FRONT

Viewed from the front, a good chest must be deep for heart and lungs to function properly. It should be neither narrow nor excessively wide. If narrow there is every likelihood of the horse plaiting, going close and hitting itself. It will appear as if both legs come out of one hole. A broad chest is frequently described as 'bosomy', and horses with this feature tend to produce a rolling motion in their faster paces. Many wide-fronted horses have their forelegs too far underneath them.

A good strong chest of a middleweight hunter.

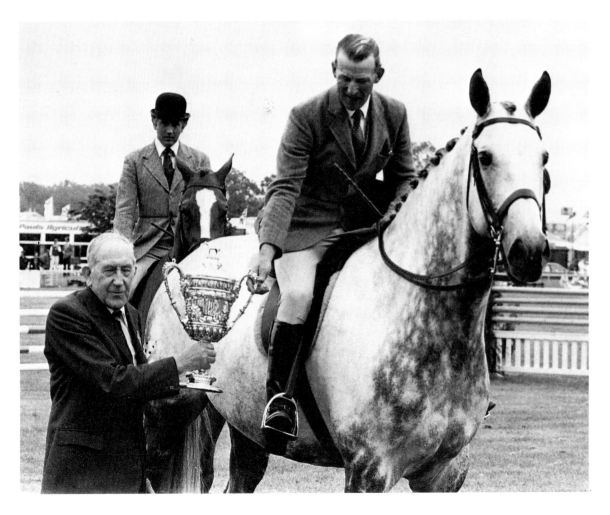

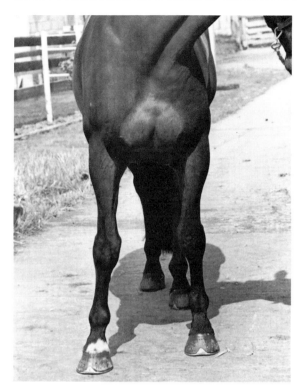

LEFT: Wide in front. (Notice also the splint on the off-fore.)

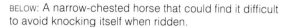

BELOW: A narrow-chested horse that could find it difficult to avoid knocking itself when ridden.

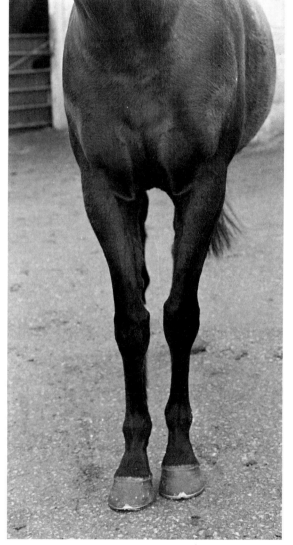

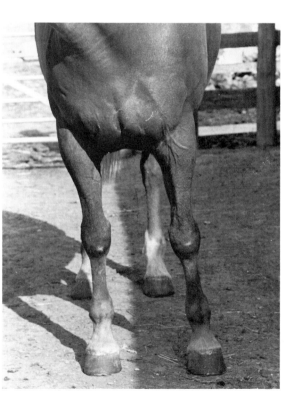

LEFT: Wide and bosomy. (This horse has scarred, broken knees.)

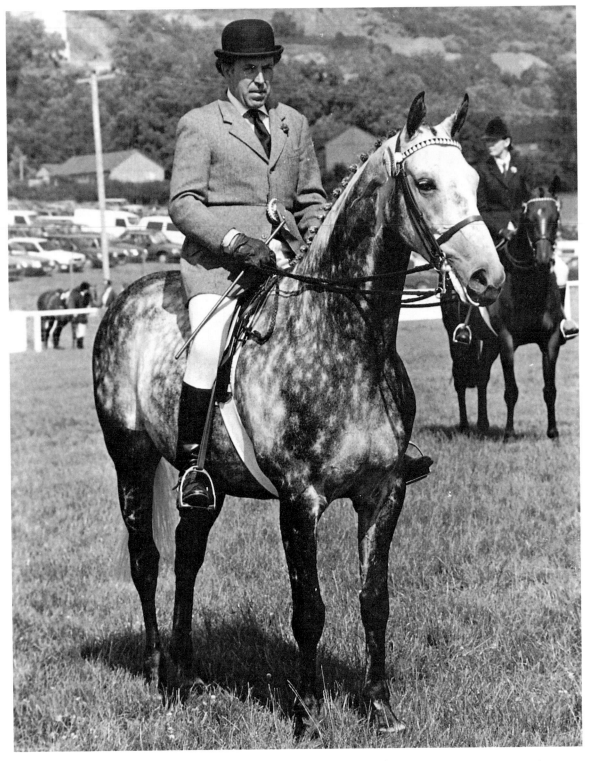

A champion hack with a front to match.

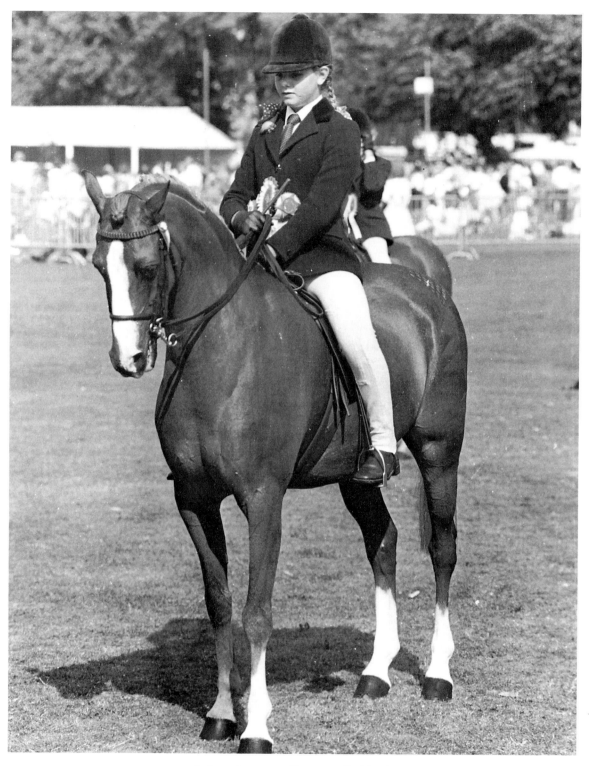

A champion pony with an excellent front.

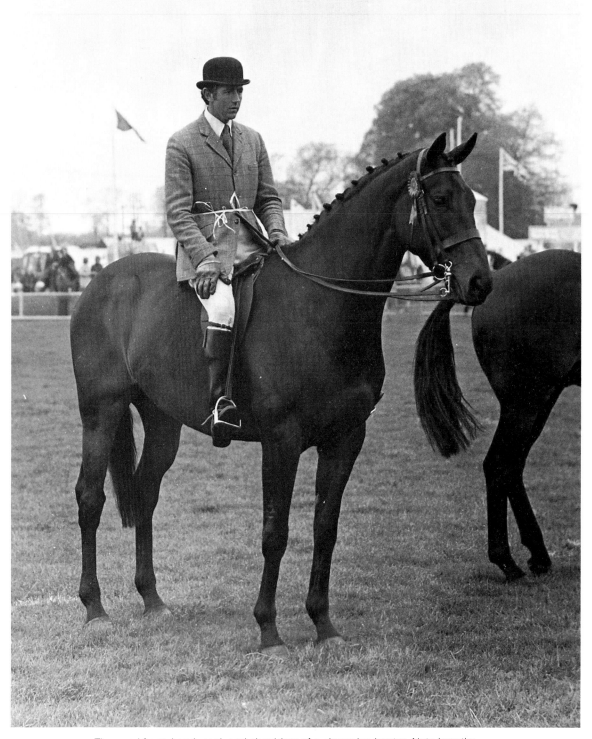

The good front, head, neck and shoulders of a champion hunter. Note how the saddle sits well behind the shoulder – no fear of the saddle or rider slipping forward on this animal.

SHOULDERS AND WITHERS

SHOULDERS

Sloping shoulders are important. They give a horse what is termed 'length of rein and a good front' or 'plenty in front of the saddle'. Good shoulders help the rider to sit in the right place, and to carry the rider's weight correctly.

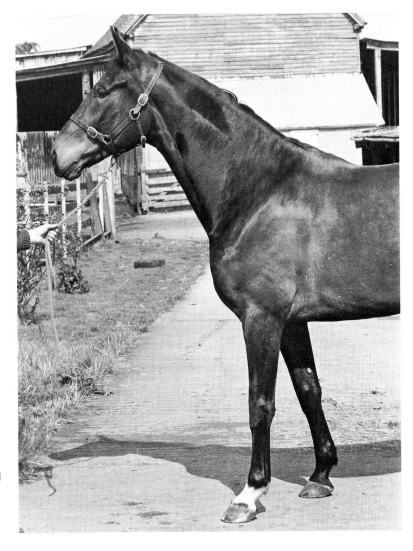

An excellent example of a correct shoulder – long and well-sloped back. In theory, the more sloping the shoulder, the better the movement and ride.

Two examples of common, coarse shoulders that would tend to make their owners moderate movers. The shoulders of both these animals run into short, thick necks. Badly positioned shoulders give uncomfortable rides; also, saddles do not stay in the right place and horses thus endowed usually go on their forehand.

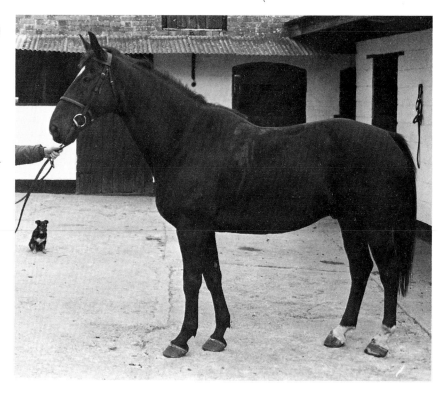

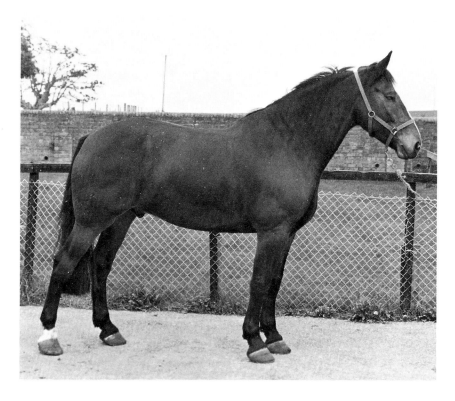

WITHERS

A correct wither should be pronounced and well defined. At maturity it should be level with the top of the quarters. Flat withers allow the saddle to slide forward and are often seen in ponies and cobs.

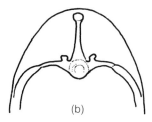

ABOVE: Withers. **(a)** Cross-section through good wither. **(b)** Cross-section through under-developed wither and loaded shoulder.

RIGHT: This horse has a quality, well-defined wither. It is, however, lower in front than behind and would therefore give a downhill ride.

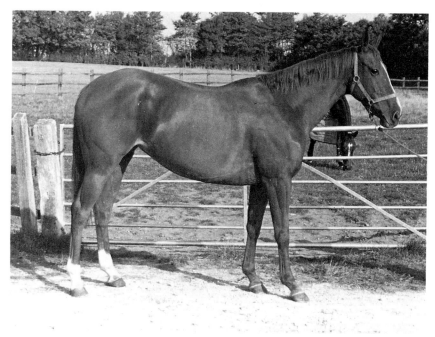

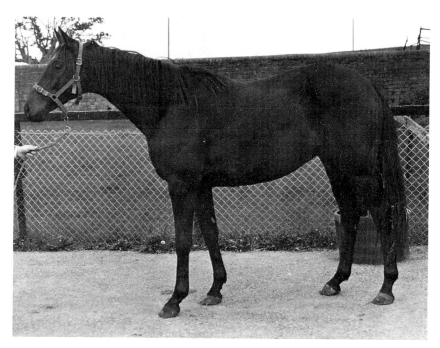

Another horse which is lower in front than behind. Nevertheless he has a lovely head, a good length of rein and a good shoulder.

This horse is slightly higher
in front than behind and his
head and neck are set on
high. This horse would find
it relatively easy to carry
himself lightly and correctly.
A very good, workmanlike
horse.

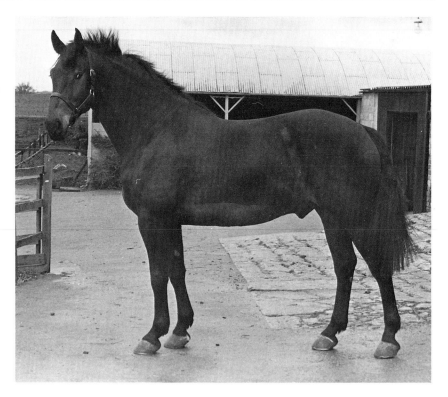

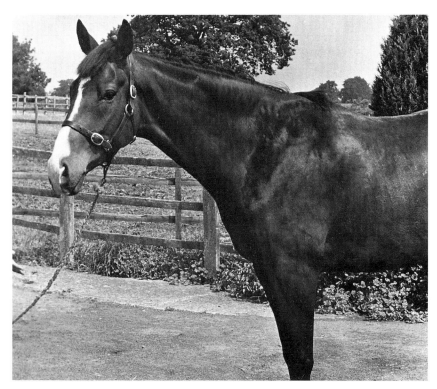

Despite a lovely head and
neck, this horse's neck
comes out of the withers
long and low. The shoulder
is very straight.

Flat withers together with a straight shoulder that is loaded. Note also how straight and upright this horse is in its forelegs. Loaded shoulders are wide and uncomfortable and often interfere with the movement of the horse.

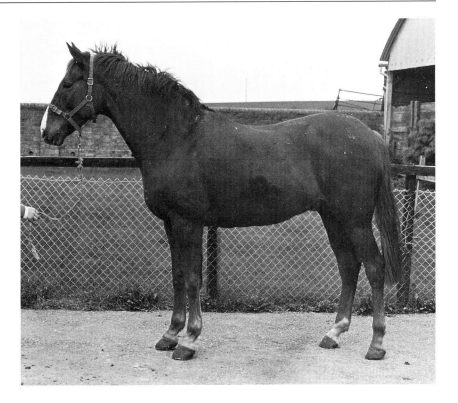

Close-up of loaded shoulders. The heaviness and extra width hinders movement and makes saddle-fitting difficult. Loaded shoulders can be uncomfortably wide to sit on.

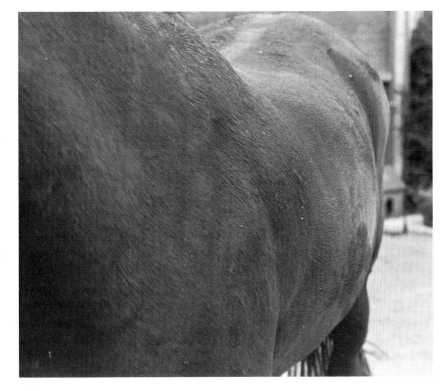

NECK

The angle at which the shoulder blade is set can create an optical illusion of shortening or lengthening the neck. The length of neck (along topline) is the same in both drawings, yet the horse with the more upright shoulder blade appears to have the longer neck.

The horse's neck is the balancing pole of his conformation. It is also the part which determines whether the animal is attractive or not. A very short neck is not desirable in the ridden horse as it is usually accompanied by a straight shoulder and can give the rider a feeling of insecurity as there is nothing in front of him. An average length of neck with a nice arch is ideal. A short, upside-down neck, known as a ewe neck, is both unattractive and universally disliked.

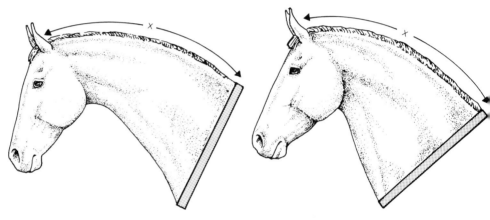

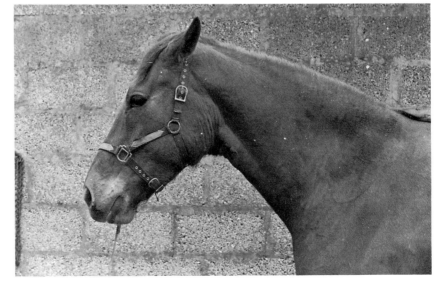

An extremely short-necked horse; moreover, the neck is badly set on to the head. A short, thick neck makes it hard for the animal to flex. Many cob-type animals have this fault, which can make them short in front to ride and strong to hold. This horse has a thick fleshy throat that could easily interfere with respiratory freedom. He also has a very prominent parotid gland.

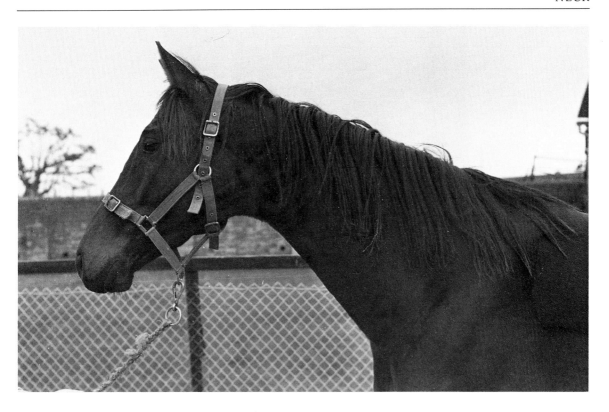

ABOVE: A long, lean neck more typical of the thoroughbred type. Very clean through the gullet and jawline.

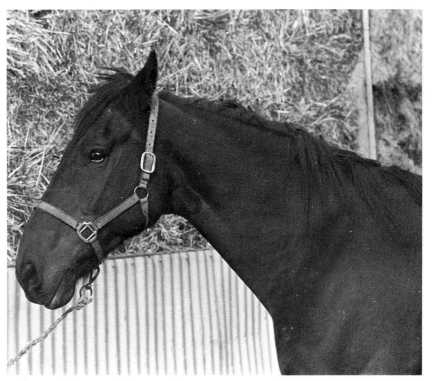

An average neck that could be improved with feeding and work. It comes out of the wither rather low.

A lovely quality head running correctly into a well-developed, muscled-up neck.

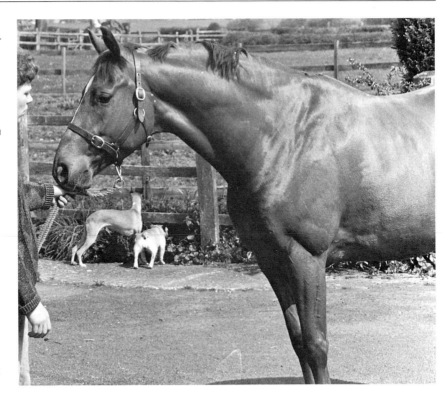

BELOW: Peacocky. This horse's head is set badly on to an almost upside-down neck (ewe-neck). The neck runs down into an upright shoulder, which is a shame as the face is attractive. No amount of condition or schooling could put this animal right for competition work.

BELOW, RIGHT: Another poor-fronted horse, with a straight shoulder and a short ewe-neck. Note the increase of muscle on the underside of the neck and the gross lack of topline. Would be very short in front to ride.

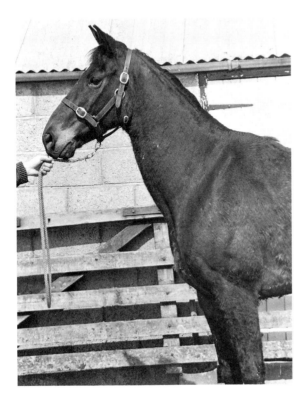

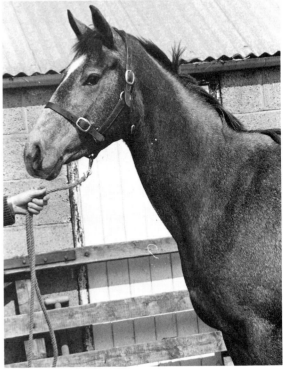

HEAD

The ideal head is in proportion to the size of the animal. A good strong jaw-line, with ample room between the two sides of the jaw bone, is required for the respiratory tract to operate efficiently. It is not desirable to have too pretty a head on a hunter, nor a plain head on a quality animal. The head and expression often reveal much about the temperament of the horse.

Small head in relation to body size.

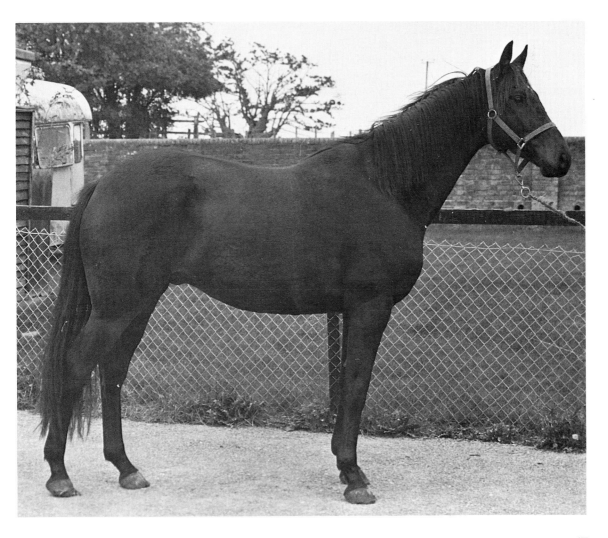

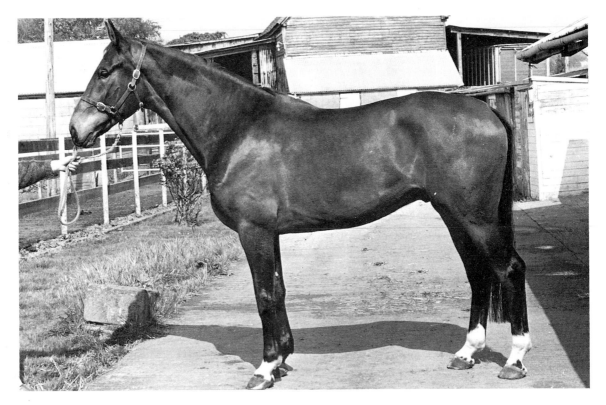

ABOVE: Head and body in proportion.

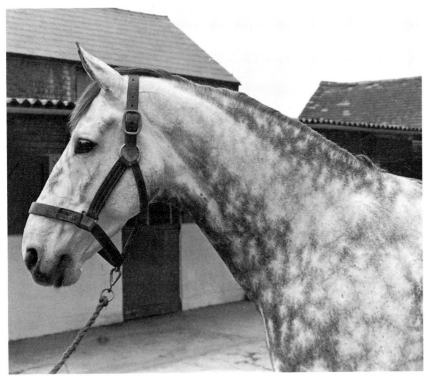

LEFT: A wonderful outlook with a fine, clean jawline, belonging to an intelligent heavyweight hunter. Lovely, big, bold eye. The head is a little on the long side but it is well put on to the neck, which should always be much longer on the topside. The whole neck should be well arched and muscled along the topline. The fit horse is often judged by the hardness of the muscle on the neck.

OPPOSITE: A good, workmanlike head of a cob, showing lots of character and a big, bold, bright eye, large wide muzzle and jaw, but relatively short in the head.

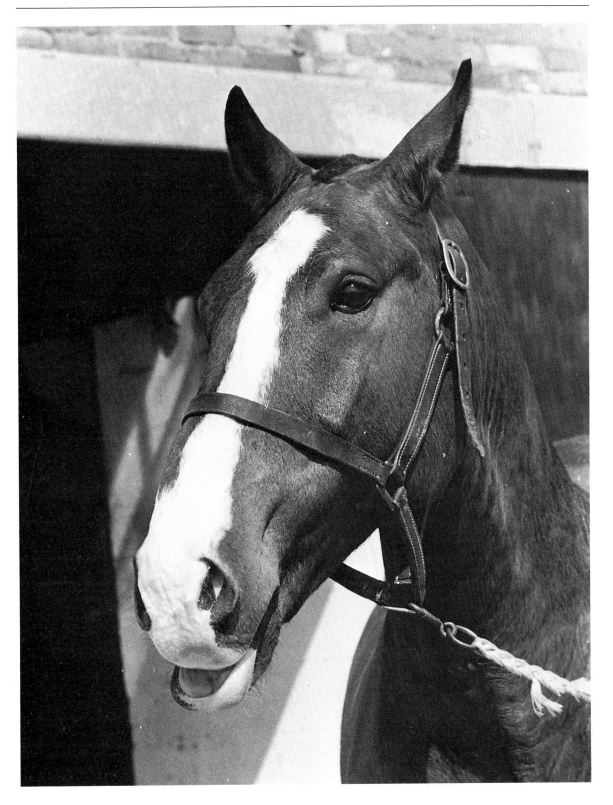

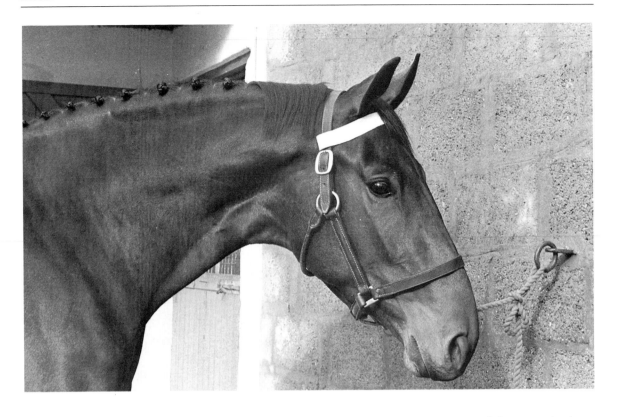

ABOVE: A fine example of a quality middleweight hunter's head, beautifully set on to its neck. The head is very clean cut with good bone structure, and the nose is full, fine and sensitive. The eyes are large and bold, giving an impression of intelligence and honesty.

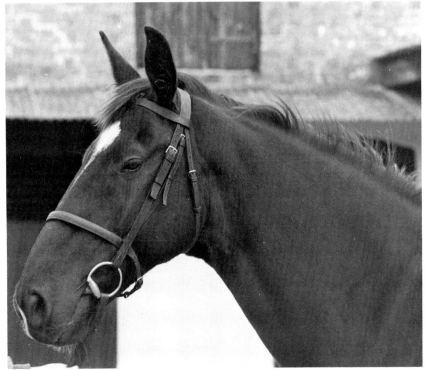

A long, narrow head with average width between the eyes. The eyes are not over-generous (i.e. on the small side) but the nostrils are nice and open. The ears are of average size. The head is not particularly well set on to the neck being thick through the gullet.

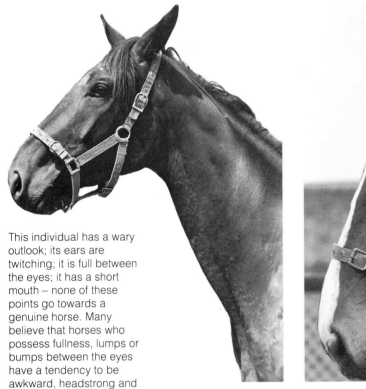

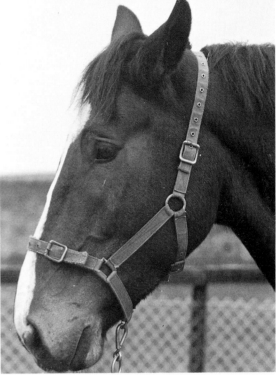

This individual has a wary outlook; its ears are twitching; it is full between the eyes; it has a short mouth – none of these points go towards a genuine horse. Many believe that horses who possess fullness, lumps or bumps between the eyes have a tendency to be awkward, headstrong and generally unco-operative.

ABOVE, RIGHT: A plain, almost 'fiddle-headed' horse with a large jaw bone. This horse would find it difficult to flex at the poll. It has a small, mean eye with average-sized ears and a slight bump between its eyes.

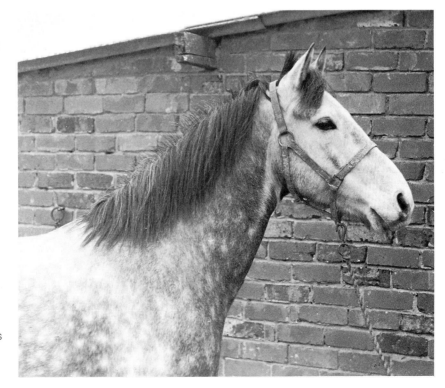

This horse has a sharp outlook and a good eye. It is thick through the gullet, which can make flexing difficult.

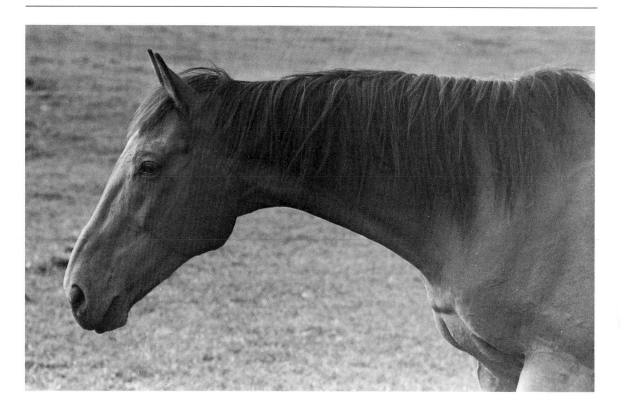

ABOVE: Lean head and neck of an old horse, in this case an eighteen-year-old thoroughbred. Notice also the straight shoulder.

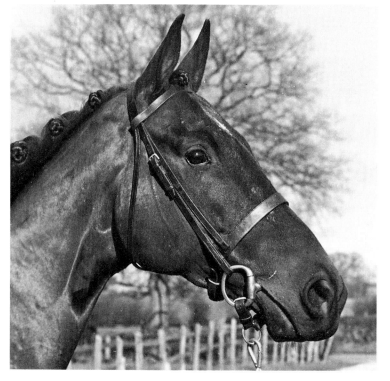

Head of a thoroughbred with a very good outlook and presence.

The cheeky face of a common-bred pony. It has a large white blaze – many would call it 'bald-faced'.

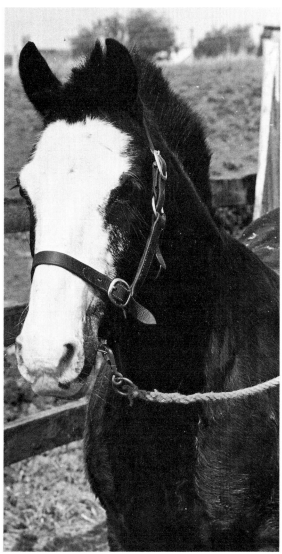

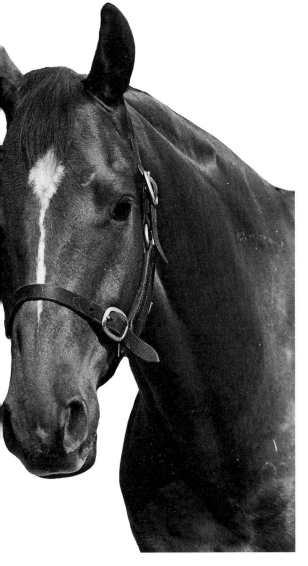

The quality head of a well-bred animal – a thoroughbred x Argentinian polo pony, who became a champion small show hunter. The head is fine, clean cut, with good bone structure, and of a size that suits the animal. The face shows a lovely, calm expression and there is considerable width between the eyes.

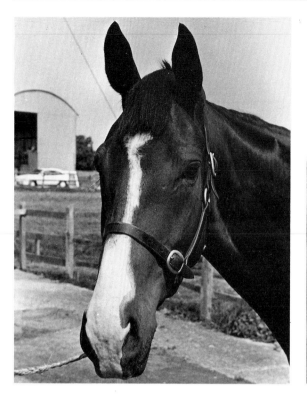

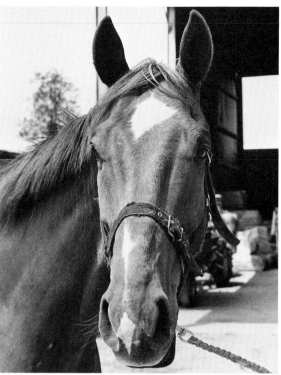

ABOVE: A lovely, honest, quality hunter's head showing an attractive narrow white blaze with a white nose.

ABOVE, RIGHT: A large white star with a snip on the muzzle.

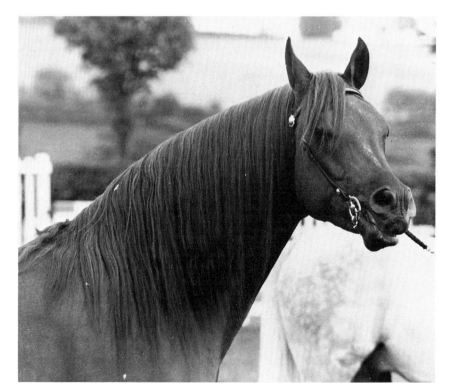

A dished face of a champion Arab, showing also natural mane and curly ears.

NOSTRILS

These are important because they are part of the breathing apparatus. Narrow, coarse nostrils are to be avoided, especially on a hunter. A good nostril should be fine and sensitive, yet open and full-looking. Nostrils can make or break the expression of a horse.

The noble head of a Shire, showing a Roman nose, bald face (i.e. white from the forehead, down the front of the face and extending towards the mouth) and small nostrils.

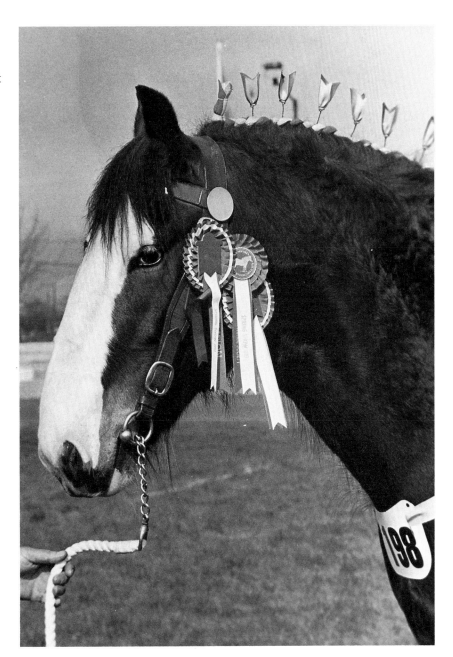

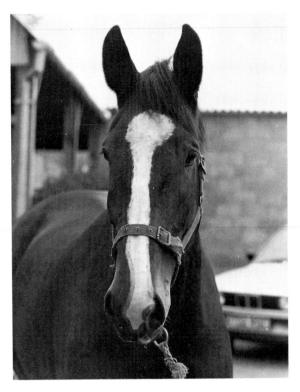

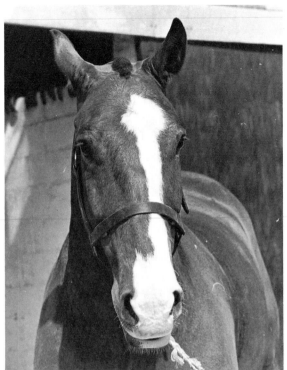

ABOVE: White blaze on a common head, which is narrow between the eyes for a big horse. The nostrils are nice and large and open.

ABOVE RIGHT: Unusual white blaze on a cob. Nice large, open nostrils.

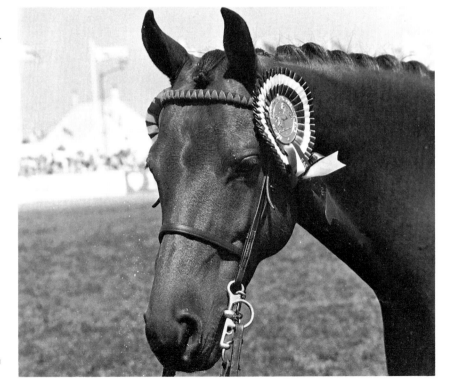

Pretty head of a champion show pony. The head is short with nice open nostrils. There is good width between the eyes.

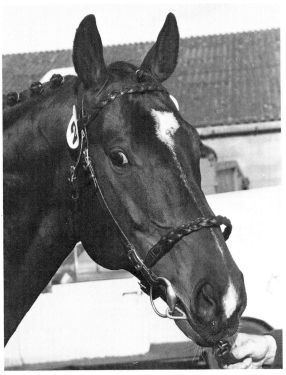

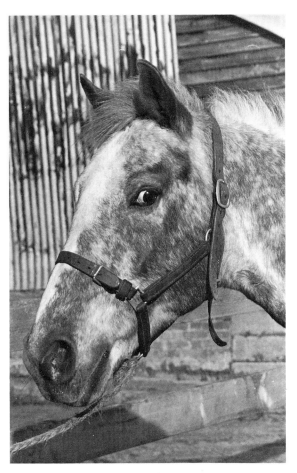

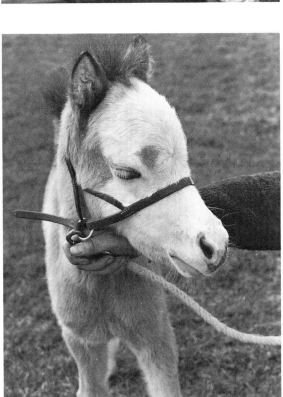

ABOVE LEFT: Large white star running into a very narrow stripe and snip. This horse is naturally showing the white of its eye and it is quite thick through the jaw bone.

ABOVE: Head of a common pony who naturally shows the white of its eye. It has good, large, open nostrils and an excellent long mouth. This individual is a really genuine old pony aged sixteen years.

The dished face of a Welsh Mountain pony foal.

EYES

Everyone likes to see large, bold eyes set well apart; such features usually go hand in hand with a good honest temperament. Eyes which lie close together, or which are small and narrow can often indicate an indifferent temperament, especially if accompanied by a bump on the forehead. This latter characteristic is not only unsightly but also can imply an ungenerous temperament.

Horses will show the whites of their eyes in fear and bad temper, but many are born with natural white pigmentation, or wall eye.

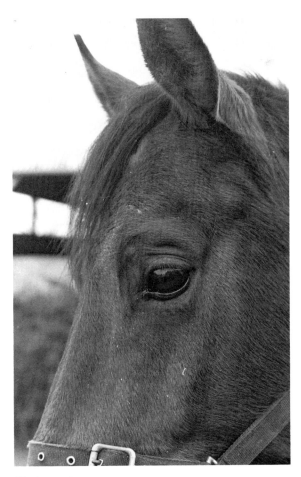

Kind, genuine eye.

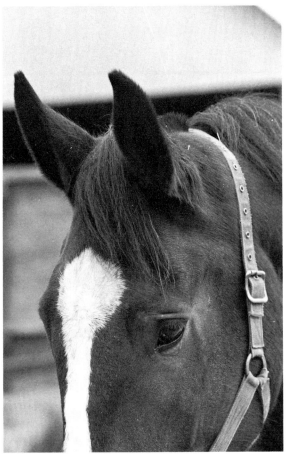

Small, narrow eye.

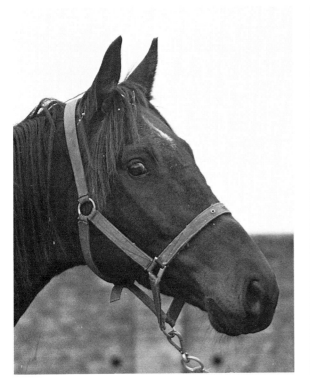

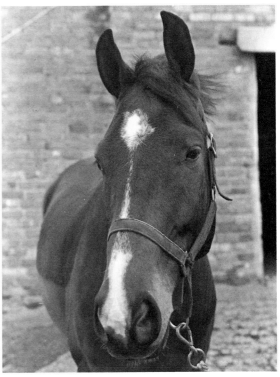

ABOVE: Eyes set well apart.

ABOVE, LEFT: Alert eye just showing the white.

A natural excess of white pigmentation.

EARS

The size and shape of the ears can alter the horse's expression. Ears vary from the small, neat pony ears to the large, plain, common, badly set on type.

The horse's temperament is often revealed by its ears: ears which are small and set close together may indicate a difficult, sharp nature. Ears that are laid flat back are usually a sign of bad temper. Those that are readily pricked show a keener outlook and are nicer to sit behind as they give the rider confidence.

Many show people favour small neat ears, but I personally prefer large generous ones. The racing fraternity do not object to large, loppy ears. Ideally the ears should be in proportion to the animal. In winter, woolly-coated ears can be clipped and trimmed to improve their appearance.

In the past, ears were often cut in various ways as a means of identification. Thankfully this practice has died out.

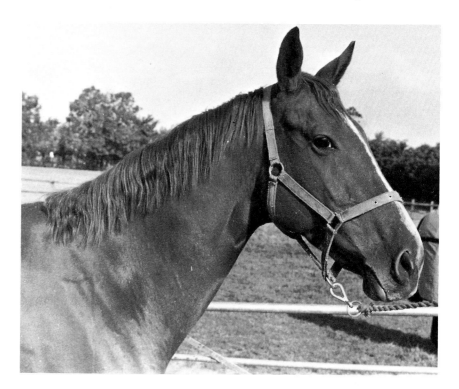

Large ears in proportion to the horse.

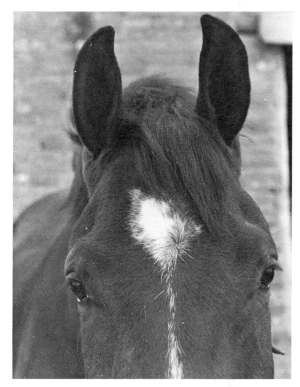

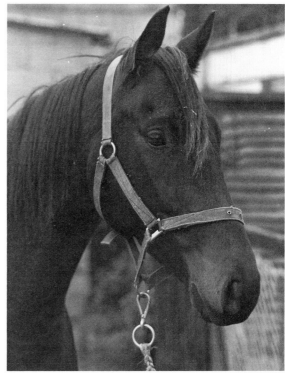

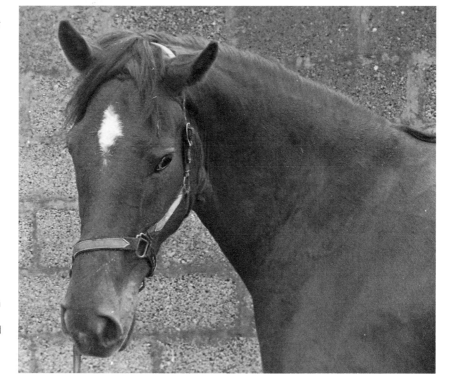

ABOVE: Slightly curly ears often show lots of character and are frequently seen in Arabs. Ears of this shape can add to the beauty of a good head.

ABOVE, RIGHT: Quality ears, untrimmed, on a nice intelligent head.

Loppy ears are those which are carried out sideways. They are usually associated with genuine horses, and many thoroughbreds are seen with them.

THE TEETH AND AGEING

The development of teeth in the horse is regular, and to a great extent gives a reliable indication of the animal's age. Every horseman should know the different characteristics of teeth from birth to nine years old, at least. Studying the relevant diagrams will help but there is no substitute for practical experience and 'field work' under the eye of an expert.

Like us, the horse has two sets of teeth: temporary teeth (milk teeth) and permanent teeth. The milk teeth are usually smaller, smoother and whiter than their permanent replacements. 'Adult' teeth are larger, stronger and yellowish in colour.

The horse has six incisor (biting) teeth in the upper jaw, and six in the lower jaw. The middle pair are called 'centrals', the next two teeth on either side are known as 'laterals', and the two outer teeth are 'corners'.

Behind the incisor teeth lie the powerful molar (cheek) teeth, whose function is to grind the horse's food. An adult horse has twenty-four permanent molars – six in each upper and lower jaw – whereas an immature animal has only twelve temporary molars.

The jaw. **(a)** Overshot – parrot-mouthed. **(b)** Undershot.

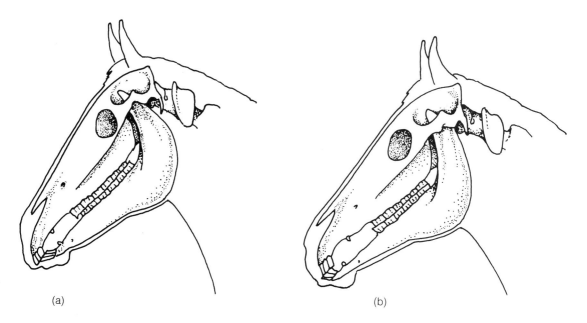

(a)   (b)

As the incisor teeth wear down with age, their changes in appearance can be used for assessing age. However, whilst such assessments can be made with reasonable accuracy up to the age of eight, thereafter they become slightly less reliable.

Around the age of nine or ten years, a brownish groove – Galvayne's groove – appears at the top of the outer surface of the upper corner incisor. Over the next ten years or so the groove continues to travel down the length of the tooth and finally disappears completely by about the age of thirty.

With advancing age the incisors become longer (hence the expression 'long in the tooth') and if viewed from the side can be seen to assume a more sloping angle.

Male horses have four additional teeth, known as tushes or canine teeth. These appear just behind the front teeth at around the age of four years and grow longer as the horse gets older. They are rarely found in mares.

Wolf teeth occasionally appear just in front of the molars in the upper jaw. They vary in size from being small and insignificant to quite large and troublesome. They can sometimes interfere with the bit and cause horses to become one-sided or fussy when ridden. To avoid problems they are best extracted.

Abnormal wear on the front teeth – i.e. worn edges, loss of enamel, discoloration – can be a sign of a crib-biter.

Cross-section through the tooth showing structure of the tooth-table when the tooth has worn down to the level indicated.

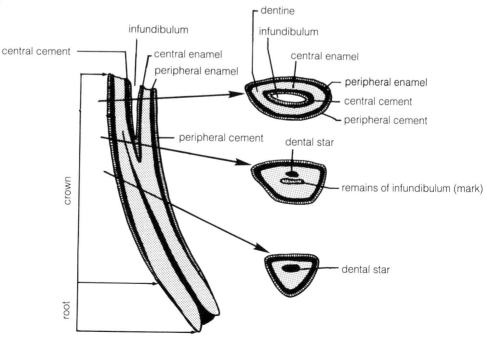

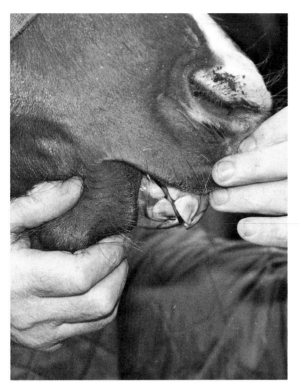

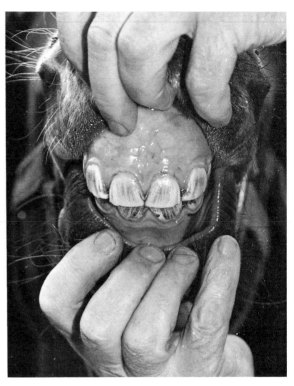

Yearling. The corner milk teeth are up, but the edges do not yet meet. At one year, all temporary teeth are through. By this time two pairs of permanent teeth, the fourth molars, have made their appearance, and the yearling therefore has sixteen molars and twelve incisors. This individual has a slight parrot mouth – i.e. the upper teeth overhang the lower teeth.

lateral temporary incisor

corner temporary incisor

central temporary incisor

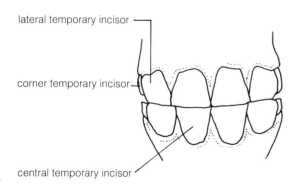

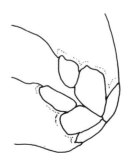

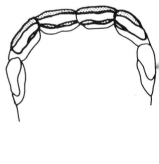

1 year old.

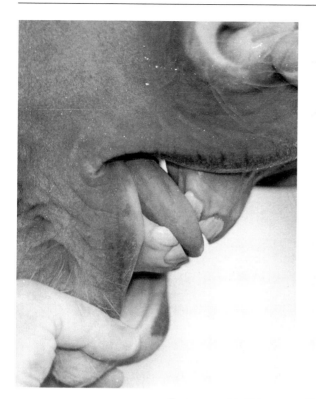
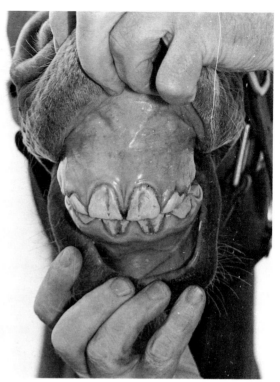

Two years old. At two years there is a full mouth of milk incisors. A two-year-old mouth can be mistaken for that of a five-year-old. However, the maturity of the animal would guide the knowledgeable person.

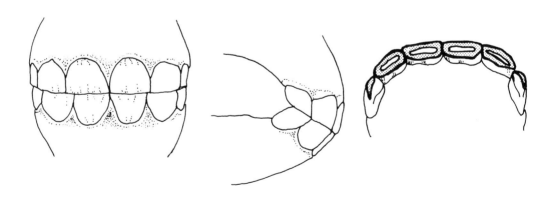

2 years old.

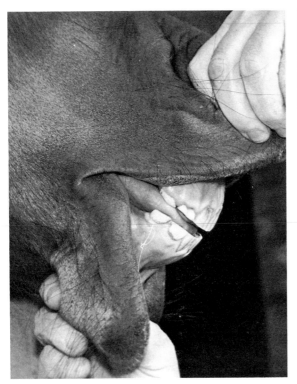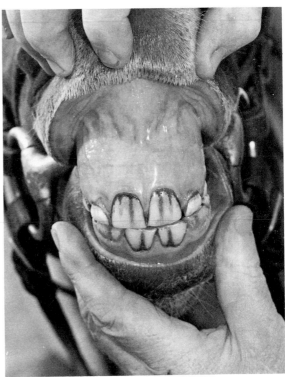

Three years old. The horse has two central adult teeth at three years. In the autumn, the milk teeth are shed and the permanent teeth come through.

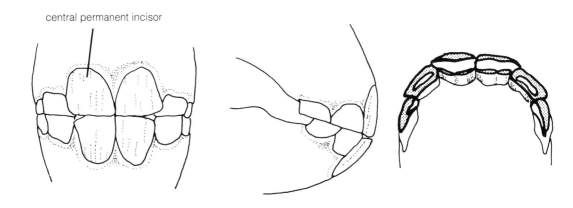

central permanent incisor

3 years old.

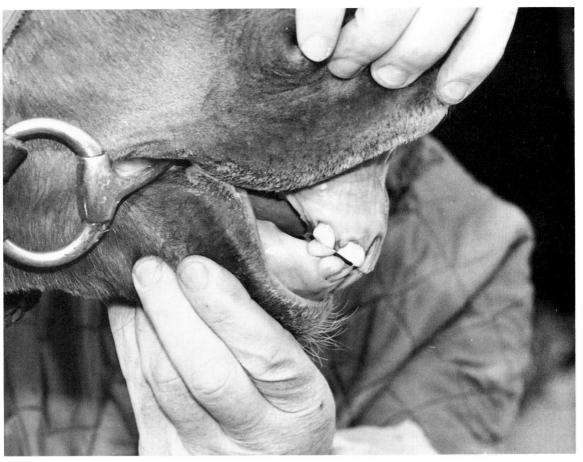

Three-and-a-half-year-old pony. When rising four the lateral teeth are in the mouth but the edges do not meet. Four pairs of adult teeth are up, but the corner milk teeth are retained.

lateral permanent incisor

central permanent incisor

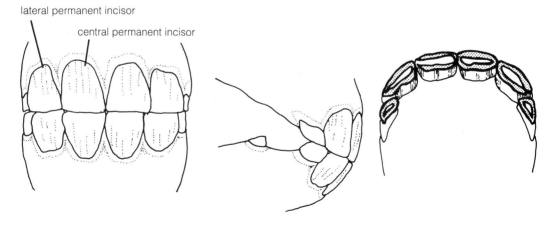

4 years old.

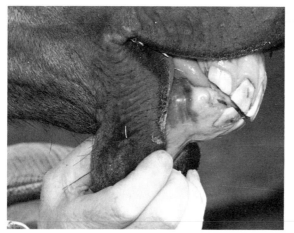

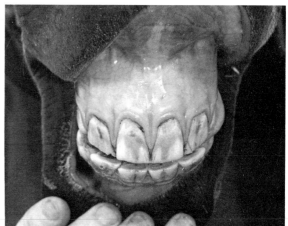

ABOVE: Five years old. There is a full mouth of horse incisors, all the edges of which meet fairly. The mouth should look more powerful than it did at four years. The teeth are fairly close and show slight signs of wear.

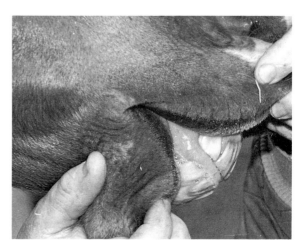

Five years old, rising six. The horse is now full-mouthed. All the incisors should meet squarely; the tooth enamel should be bright in colour.

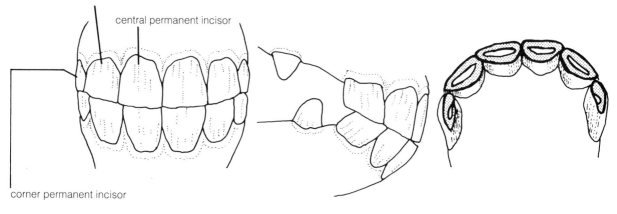

lateral permanent incisor

central permanent incisor

corner permanent incisor

5 years old.

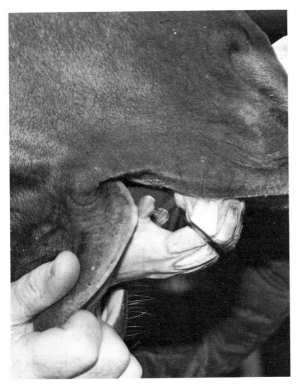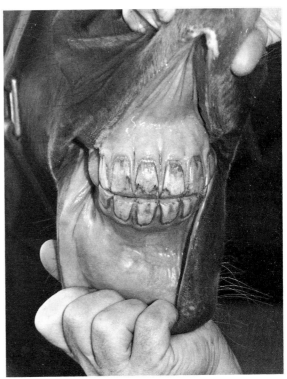

Six years old. The corner teeth look more firmly set, and their edges begin to be uneven. At six years teeth become more square on the external surfaces and look more permanent in character. When the jaw is closed, the corner teeth display considerable use. The edges of this animal's teeth are damaged from chewing, or possibly from crib-biting.

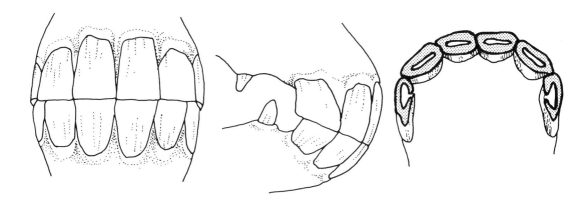

6 years old.

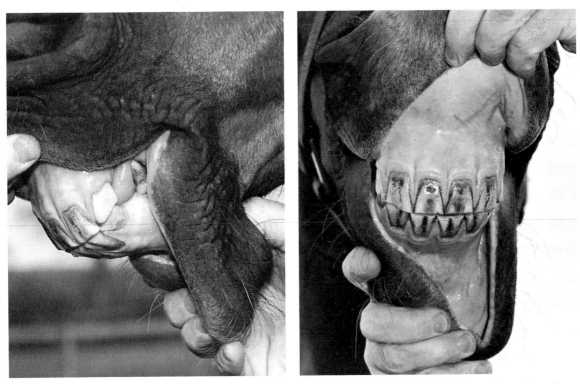

Seven years old. The corner teeth exhibit further evidence of wear. As yet there is no sign of the seven-year hook, which develops as the result of such wear.

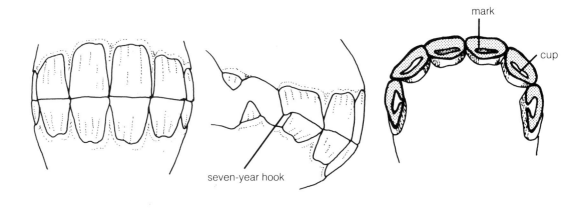

seven-year hook

mark

cup

7 years old.

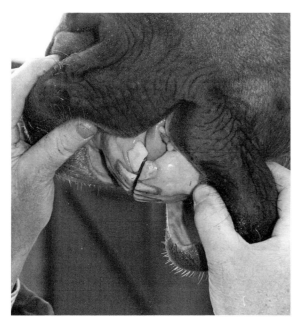
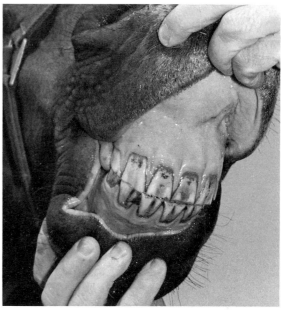

Eight years old. The seven-year hook has disappeared and at eight years the teeth are set. In geldings the tush has become square. The inside tables of the teeth are now full. At eight and over, the horse is described as 'aged'.

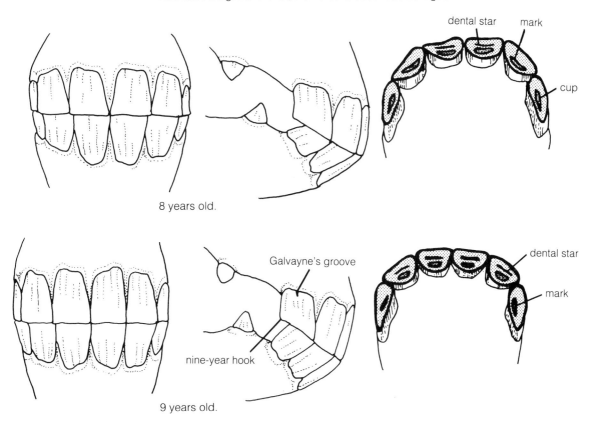

8 years old.

9 years old.

91

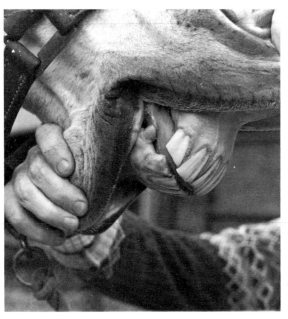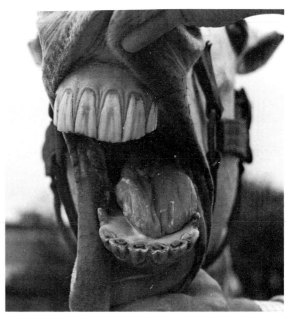

Older horse. The photographs show sets of twelve-year-old teeth. The difference is marked: they have become larger, more crowded, darker in colour, and the angle of the teeth in the jaw is more pronounced.

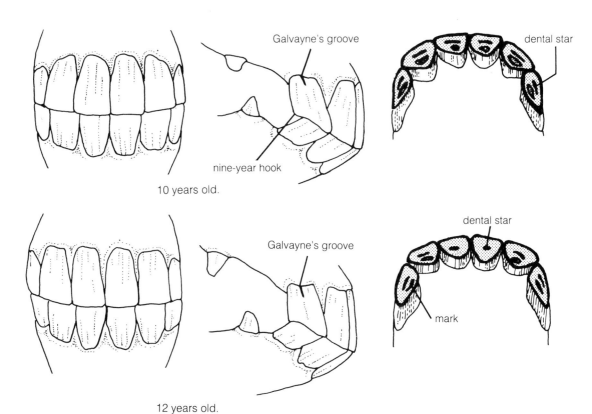

10 years old.

12 years old.

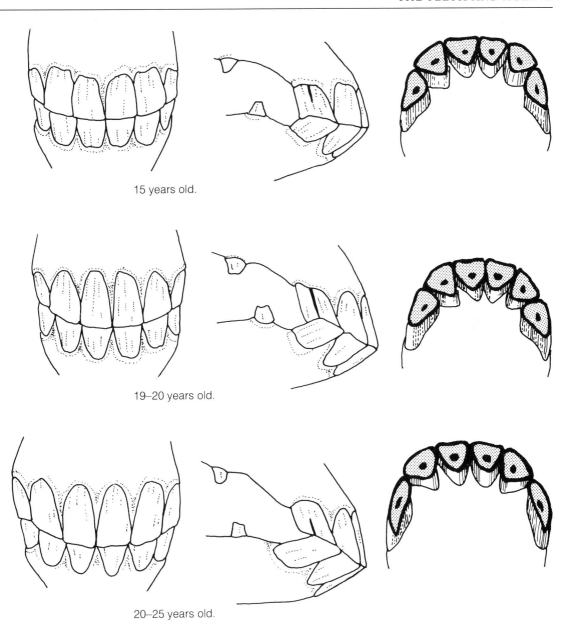

15 years old.

19–20 years old.

20–25 years old.

COLOURS
AND MARKINGS

Horses come in many different colours, with bay, brown, black, chestnut, grey and roan predominating. In general, the horse world prefers a good strong coat colour, but this is very much a matter of personal taste. Various breeds have their own distinctive colour characteristics – such as Suffolk Punches, which are always chestnut, and Haflingers, which are chestnut with a flaxen mane and tail – and breed societies lay down strict guidelines to preserve these traits.

The horseman's proverb that 'Every good horse is a good colour' may well be true, but there are some body colours that can diminsh the value of an otherwise useful horse. Chestnut mares, in particular, can suffer in this way, as can very light or white greys, or light, wishy-washy chestnuts.

Coat colour can be affected by clipping; and a horse's winter coat may be a different shade to his summer one. A dull, staring coat is a sign of ill-health.

Coat colours

Bay is possibly the most popular colour of all. Bays have black manes and tails and usually some black on the limbs; their body colour comes in various shades – light (yellowish/reddish); bright (mahogany); and dark (rich, dark brown).

Black can be a most attractive coat colour, especially when the horse is in good condition and the coat gleams. Black horses should have black points and a black muzzle.

Brown is dark brown in colour with black limbs, mane and tail. It is darker than a dark bay.

Chestnut horses come in various shades: dark, liver and light. The light types often have a flaxen mane and tail, while those of the darker chestnuts are self-colour. In some parts of the world the colour is known as 'sorrel'.

Grey is a combination of white hairs and black hairs on a dark skin. Flea-bitten greys, however, sometimes feature brown hairs in their coats, which have a speckled appearance. Dapple greys have circular patches of darker hairs growing over the body. Iron grey horses have predominantly black hairs and can be very dark indeed. Rose greys have a little chestnut or brown in the coat giving it a warm tinge. The grey's coat usually becomes lighter as the horse ages, sometimes to the point of becoming completely white.

Roan horses have a mixture of two colours (one of which is white) growing in the coat. The blue roan has a combination of black and white coat hairs with black points; the strawberry roan is chestnut and white with chestnut points; the bay roan is bay and white with black points and black on the limbs, tail and mane.

Duns can vary from being deep golden yellow to mousy in body colour but always with a black skin and black mane and tail. The blue dun is a diluted black colour; the yellow dun is a golden colour; the silver dun has a greyish hue; and the dark dun is mouse-coloured. Duns often have a black dorsal stripe running from mane to tail. The colour is more frequently seen in ponies rather than horses.

Cream horses have a cream to white body coat and the skin is pink. The eyes may also have a pinkish or bluish tinge.

Palominos are pale cream to bright gold and have lighter or silvery-coloured manes and tails. According to the British Palomino Society the coat should be 'the colour of newly minted gold'.

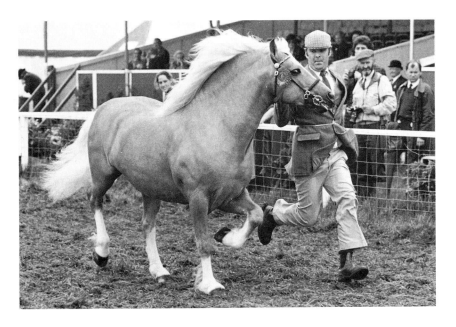

Light coloured palomino.

Dark-coated palomino.

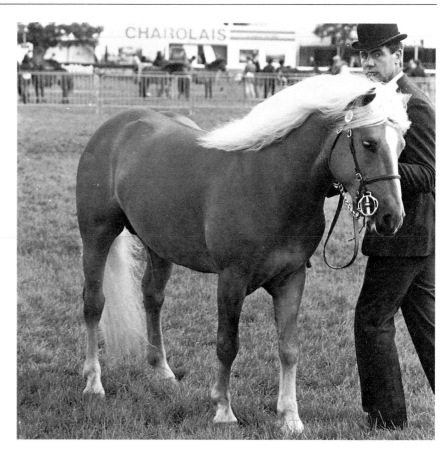

A dun pony with attractive markings, and still retaining some of its winter coat.

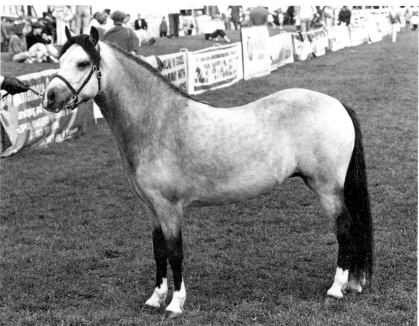

Skewbald horses have large irregular patches of white and any other colour or colours. They are most commonly brown and white.

Piebalds are a mixture of black and white in irregular patches.

Spotted horses usually have pink skin with spots of any colour on a white or light coloured background. The patterns of the spots have various names, such as leopard, blanket and snowflake. Appaloosas, which are a breed of spotted horse, have eight basic coat patterns with unlimited colour combinations.

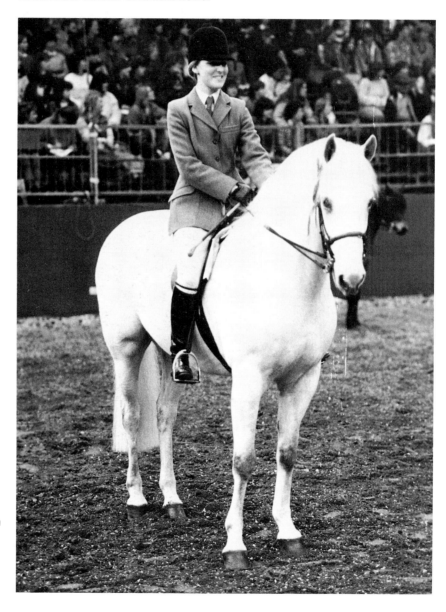

Greys vary tremendously. Many are quite dark in their younger days, and are often born black, the coat becoming lighter as the individual ages and eventually turning pure white.

Skewbald.

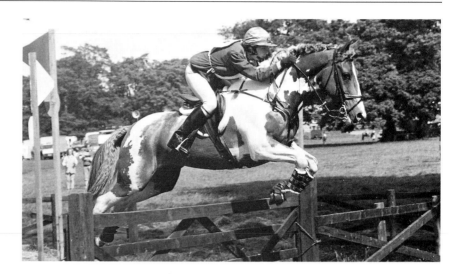

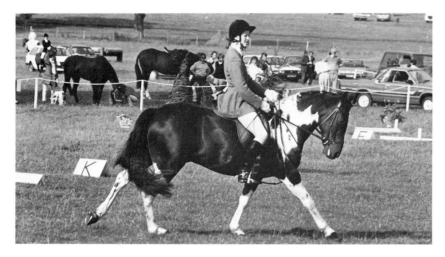

Piebald.

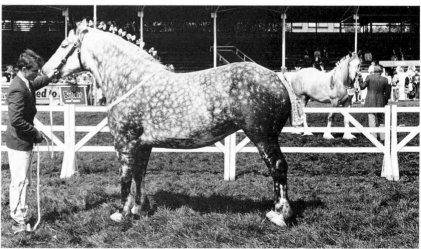

A true dapple grey – a
rocking-horse colour and a
favourite with many.

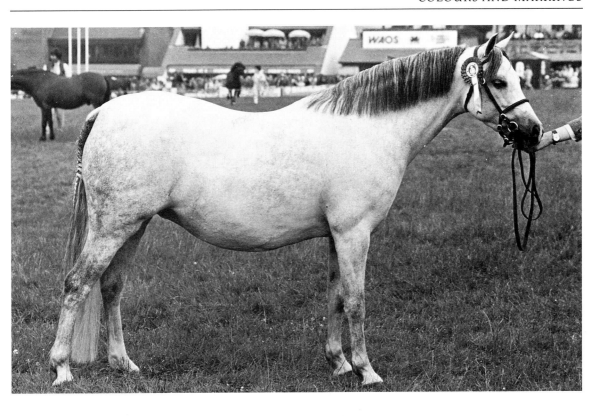

ABOVE: An average-coloured grey whose appearance is enhanced by a darker mane and tail.

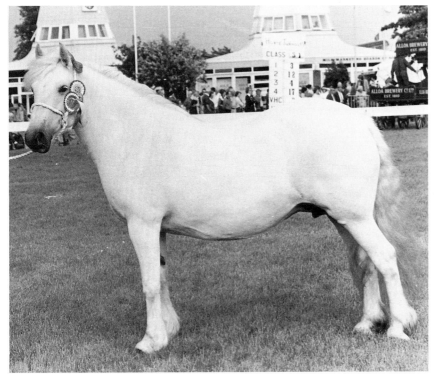

A white pony.

A flea-bitten grey Welsh
Section A pony.

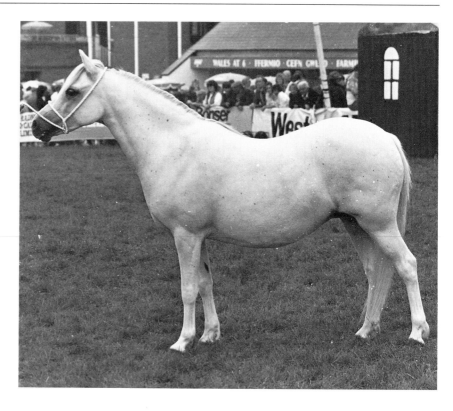

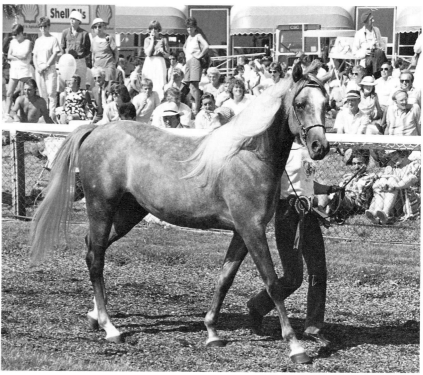

A dark grey Arab with a
lighter mane and tail.

Spotted pony.

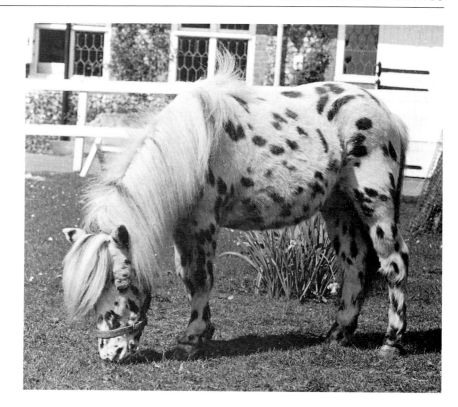

BELOW: Bay showing dappling in the coat.

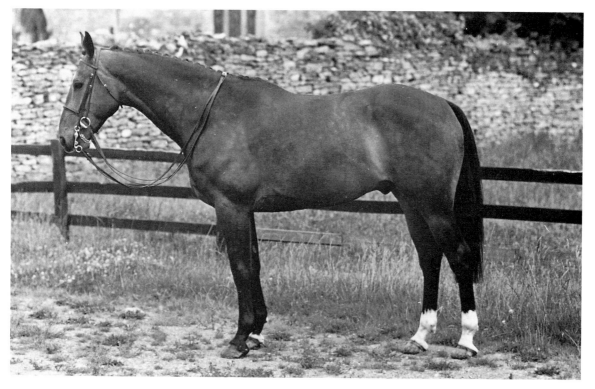

A light bay with black points.

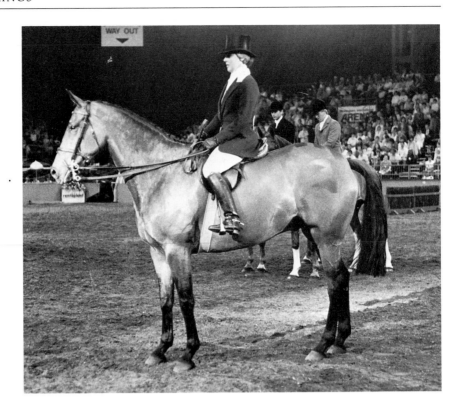

Body markings

Body markings can be an important factor in identification.

List. This is a dorsal stripe running from mane to tail. It is also known as a 'ray'.

A prophet's thumb mark is a pronounced dimple, usually found on the neck. It is considered by some to be a lucky feature; others believe it denotes a good horse.

Flesh marks. Patches where the pigment of the skin is absent.

Saddle or girth marks. These are areas of white hair caused by pressure or rubbing from ill-fitting tack.

Whorls are small areas of coat where the hair grows in the opposite direction to the rest of the coat. They are commonly found on the head, neck, chest and upper limbs.

Brands generally denote the breed and/or country of origin and are

A list, or dorsal stripe, running along the backbone.

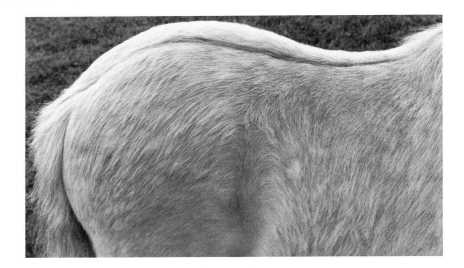

A prophet's thumb mark.

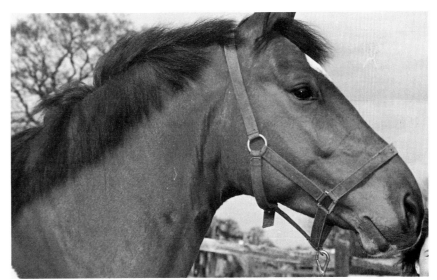

Freeze-mark placed on the neck.

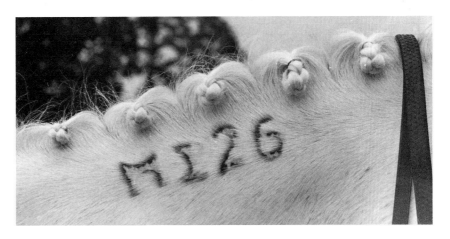

generally found on the shoulder or the quarters, but sometimes on the neck or under the saddle.

Freeze-marking is a modern method of branding which is effected by freezing the skin. Each horse is given a number which is kept on a national register and made available to the police in the event of a theft. The usual site for a freeze-mark is under the saddle, but they are also seen on the shoulders and neck.

Head markings

Blaze – a broad white marking extending down the face from the forehead.

Star – a white mark on the forehead.

Stripe or race – a narrow white mark running down the face.

Snip – a white mark between the nostrils.

White face/bald face – a large white area which includes the forehead and front of the face.

White muzzle – the term used when the whole muzzle area, including the lips and nostrils, is white.

Note: many of the above face markings are depicted in the Head section.

Leg markings

There is an old horsemen's saying about leg markings which runs thus:

> One white sock, buy him,
> Two, try him,
> Three, keep him not a day,
> Four, send him far away.

The main reason that people dislike white legs is because they have been found to suffer more from mud-fever and cracked heels, and the white feet which usually accompany them are considered by some to be not as strong as those with dark horn. However, white markings do

Two white socks.

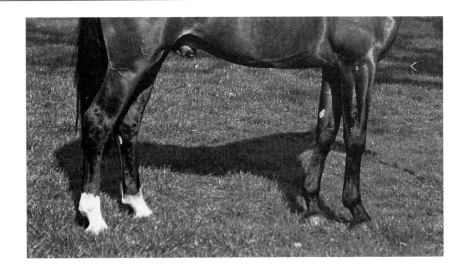

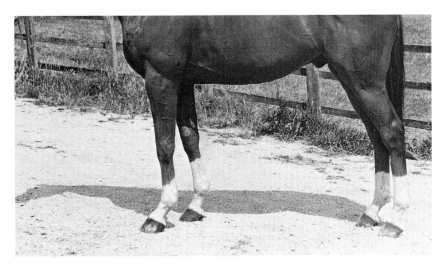

Four white stockings.

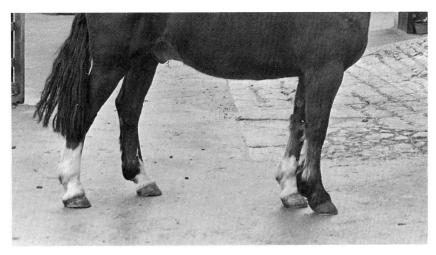

Two socks and one
stocking.

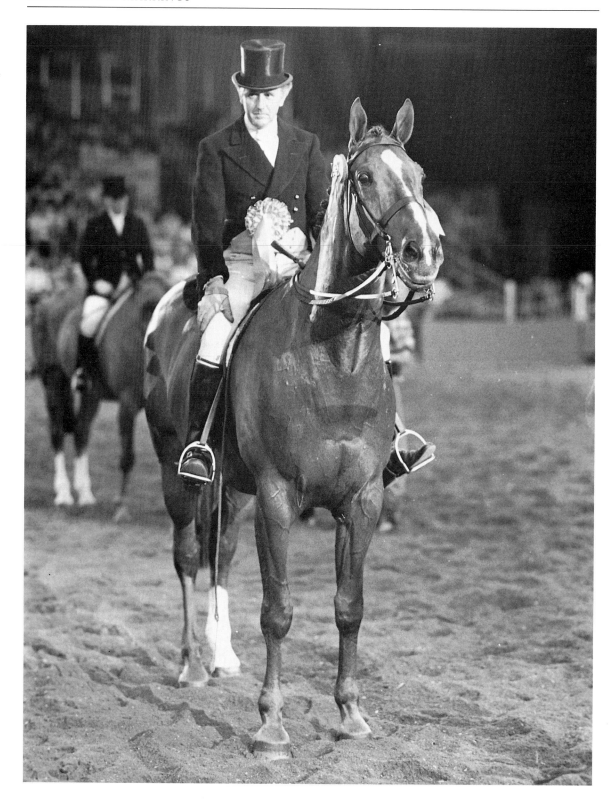

OPPOSITE: A champion hunter with one white stocking.

make horses attractive, but excessive white, to the point of making the wearer appear flashy or ugly, is frowned upon.

A sock runs from the coronet to just above the fetlock, whereas a **stocking** extends from the coronet up the leg to the knee.

Ermine marks. This term describes black spots which appear on white legs.

Feather. Copious long hair covering the lower limbs and fetlocks, seen most frequently in the heavier breeds.

Chestnuts consist of soft, horn-like tissue and are found on the inside of all four legs. They can sometimes grow quite large and become unsightly. The excess can be trimmed painlessly with a sharp knife or peeled off with the fingers.

Ergots are small horny growths found at the back of the fetlock joints. They vary in size from being barely visible in the quality animal to being quite large in the more common-bred types.

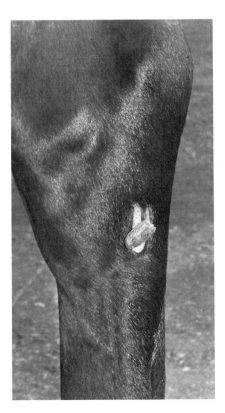 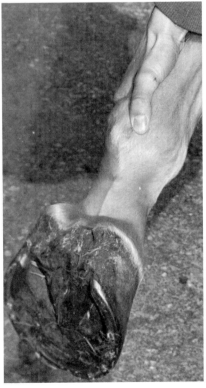

RIGHT: Hind chestnut with a piece about to be removed.

FAR RIGHT: An ergot, seen beside the thumb nail.

HORSES IN ROUGH AND SHOW CONDITION

Basic conformation cannot be altered, bad limbs especially. However, plain heads can be improved with a well-muscled neck, and poor hindquarters can look much rounder when fleshed out and muscled. Equally, over-fat animals will alter in shape through work and a correct diet. Quality, of course, is greatly improved by a summer coat and correct clipping and trimming. It is never possible, though, to 'make a silk purse out of a sow's ear.'

A quality champion hack before the start of the show season, in his winter woollies.

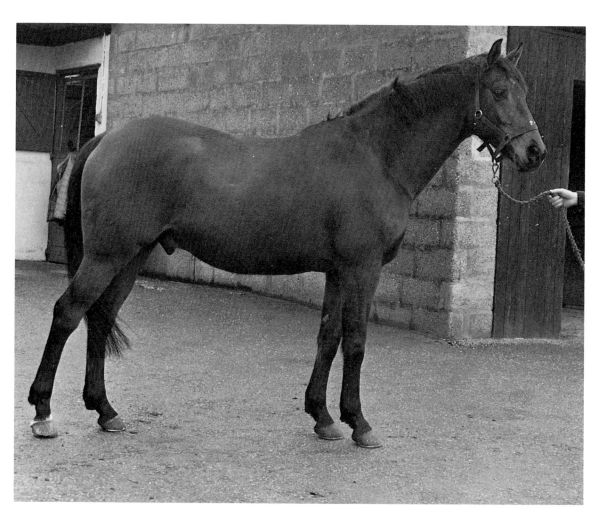

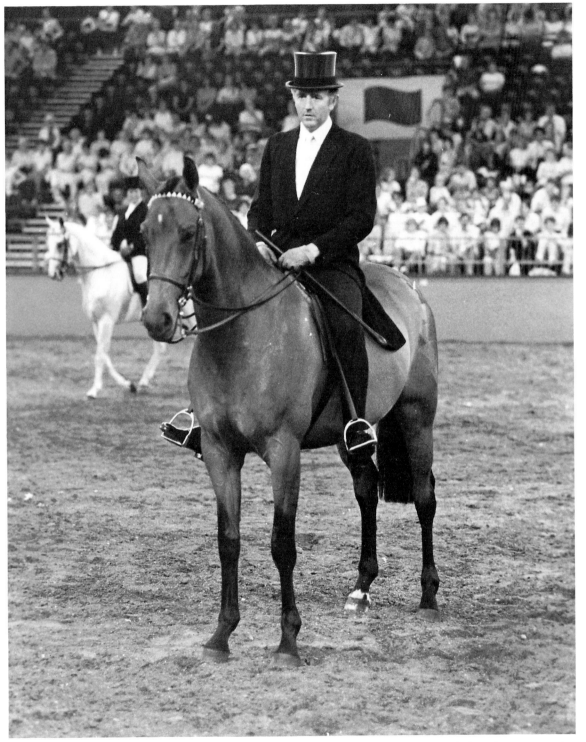

The same horse in the show ring, showing the elegance and relaxed temperament so essential in the hack.

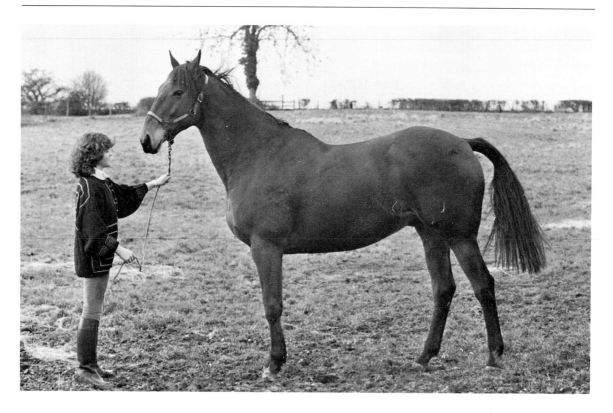

ABOVE: Middleweight hunter in February, out of work.

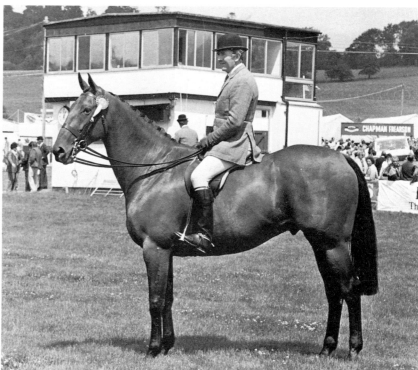

The same horse in show condition four months later, after correct work and feeding.

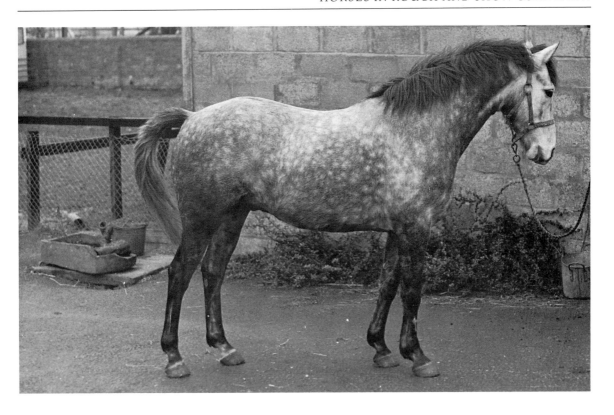

ABOVE: A show hunter pony at the end of a winter living out.

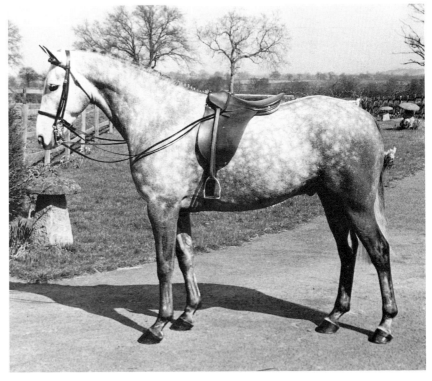

The same pony clipped and trimmed.

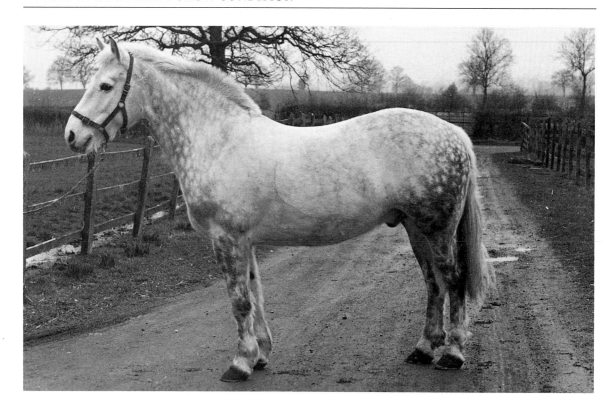

A cob in the rough . . .
. . . and ready to show. It is
often difficult for the
amateur to visualise the
potential of an animal – as
these two pictures reveal.

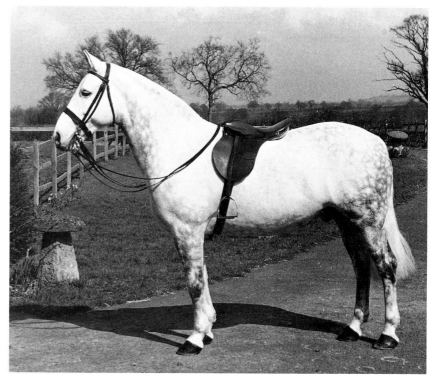

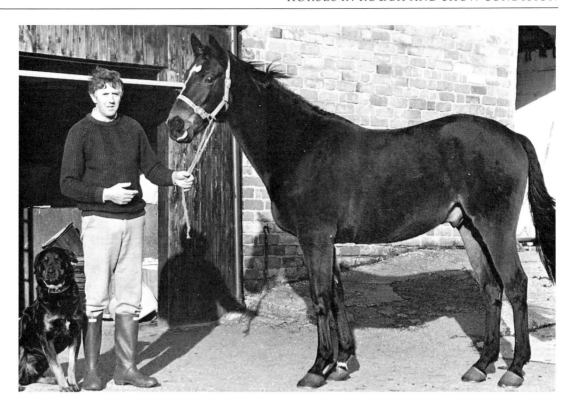

Man and horse in their working clothes.

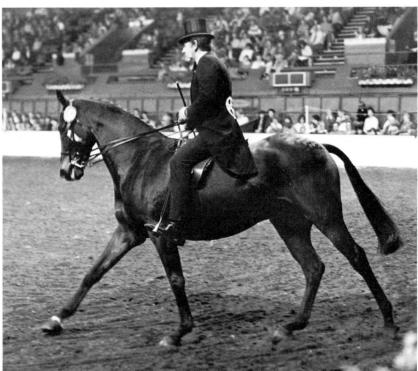

The same pair in action, winning at the Horse of the Year Show after months of preparation.

ACTION

The correctly made horse finds natural movement easy. A long, low swing to the walk is desirable. The horse's front feet should always land toe first, giving a good naturally balanced, comfortable ride.

In good action the horse moves its whole shoulder, giving full extension of the foreleg, some to the point of suspension before the foot is put to the ground.

Given room between the elbow and the ribs the animal can move really well. Good movement cannot be achieved in a horse that is tucked in at the elbows. A 'daisy-cutting' action is often the result of being restricted (tied in) at the elbows, and is seen regularly in some children's show ponies.

Elevation at the trot enables an animal to move in a graceful, floating manner.

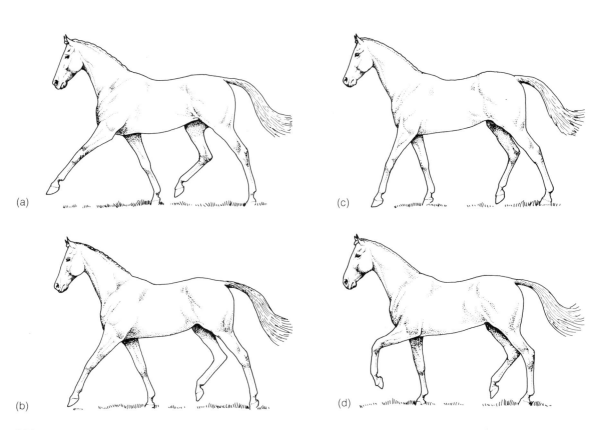

(a) (c)

(b) (d)

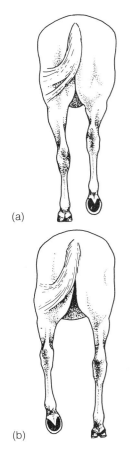

High knee action, often seen in horses that jump well, is frequently found in animals that are short-striding and straight-shouldered. High action at the trot presupposes high action at the gallop and therefore a lack of speed.

The horse's hind movement is all-important: it is impulsion from behind which produces free forward movement. The hock should always come well underneath the body to lighten the forehand. Thus animals which are allowed to get on to their forehands find it difficult to move correctly and to carry weight.

Occasionally extravagant action in front is accompanied by poor action at the back, with the horse leaving its hind legs out behind its body. This is both unsightly and not favoured.

When assessing a horse's action in hand, the horse must be walked away and trotted back in a straight line. A good striding walk is a great asset, and a horse which walks well with free movement is invariably a good horse. Many adhere to the maxim: 'A good walker, a good galloper.'

At the walk the imprints of the hind feet should overreach the imprints of the fore feet.

Remember: good action relates to good conformation, and good action goes with soundness.

Horses should move straight both in front and behind. Young, immature and unfit animals often move less than straight due to their lack of strength. In such cases the action usually improves as they become fitter, older and stronger.

Faulty action includes any form of unsoundness.

Stilted or short strides are usually the result of upright pasterns.

Hind leg movement. **(a)** Moving straight. **(b)** Moving wide, slightly bow-legged.

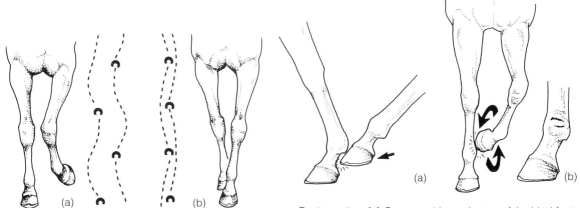

Foreleg movement. **(a)** Dishing. **(b)** Plaiting.

Faulty action. **(a)** Over-reaching – the toe of the hind foot strikes the front heel. **(b)** Brushing – the front foot strikes the inside of the opposite front leg.

If a horse or pony throws its feet out sideways at any gait it is called 'dishing'. Horses that dish are liable to strains and splints.

Animals that plait are those that cross one foot over in front of another, either behind or in front. Plaiting (or lacing) is regarded as a bad fault due to the possibility of injury.

The dragging of hind toes points to some form of hock trouble, either forming or actually present.

Interfering and brushing occurs when one joint (usually the fetlock) knocks against another, sometimes breaking the skin and ultimately enlarging the affected joint. Such problems are the result of bad conformation and are frequently seen in narrow-chested, base narrow horses. Animals with this problem can be difficult to keep sound, especially in the hunting field when they get tired. Badly shaped feet and poor shoeing can add to the cause of brushing.

Speedy cutting is a serious form of brushing which often leads to injury below the knee or hock. Horses with this problem require careful shoeing and should wear special boots for protection. Speedy cutting is caused by close, peculiar movement.

Extended trot of a champion dressage horse, on this occasion competing in a show hunter class at the Royal Show. The extended trot of a dressage horse should be powerful but with a soft round outline. In the extended paces the rider concentrates on the driving effect of the hind legs. The horse should extend its whole form, carrying its head lower.

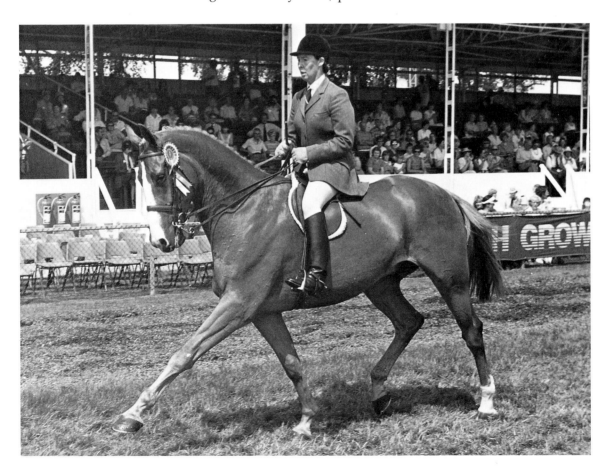

Olympic champion Reiner Klimke performing flying changes across the diagonal of the dressage arena.

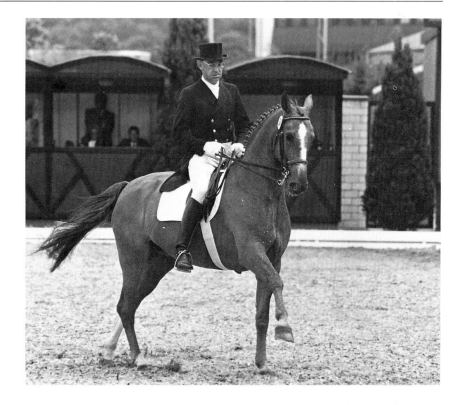

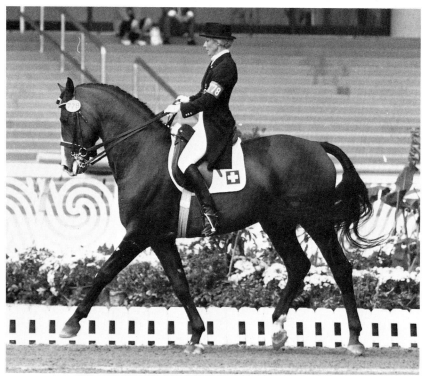

Christine Stuckelberger on Gaugin de Lully competing in the Seoul Olympics. The pair are commencing a half-pass in trot.

117

The champion middleweight hunter, Elite, showing good balance and moving freely forward in a collected canter.

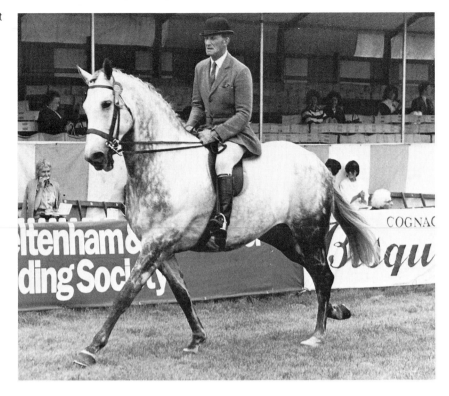

BELOW: Freeway, champion hunter at the Royal International, covering the ground while maintaining good natural balance in an extended canter.

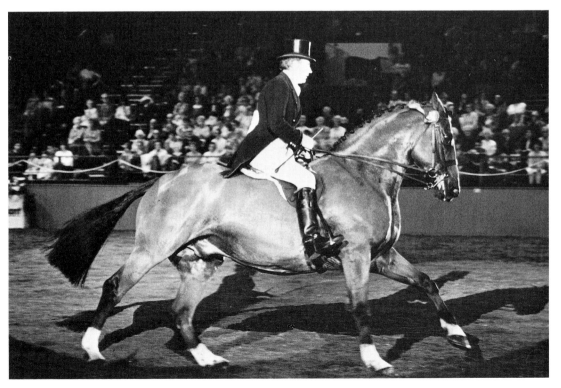

Champion middleweight, Carnival King, at full gallop. Note the extended flexion in the foreleg. The gallop is essentially an extended gait in which the horse stretches himself to the utmost.

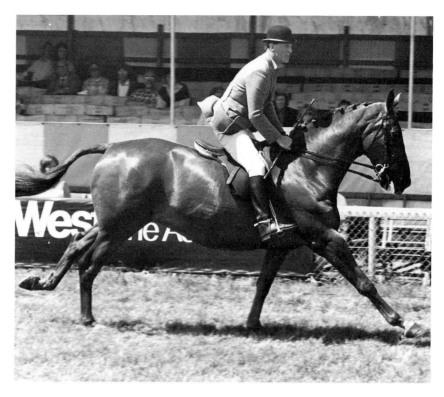

BELOW: Tomadachi, many times champion show hack, showing a long, low action at the walk. In walk the horse has never less than two legs in support at the same time. There is no moment of suspension when all four legs are off the ground. The walk should have a swing to it, in which head and neck play an important part.

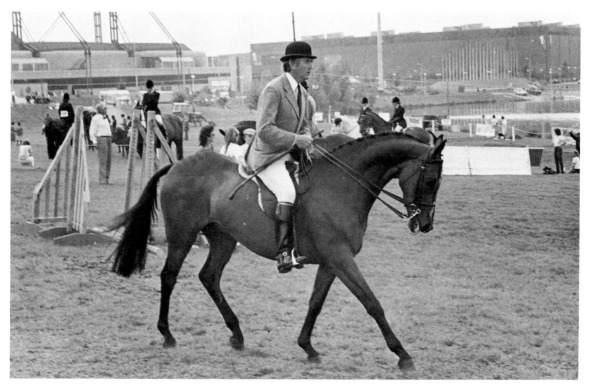

A young horse being trotted up in hand. It has a nice light action using both its quarters and shoulders with a natural flick of the toe. In the trot the horse goes naturally off his hocks and should be light in his forehand, carrying his head high.

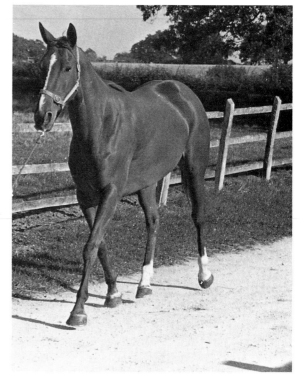

BELOW: Moving perfectly straight in front and behind.

BELOW, RIGHT: This horse is moving well and straight in front but note the crossing behind, which would make it prone to brushing.

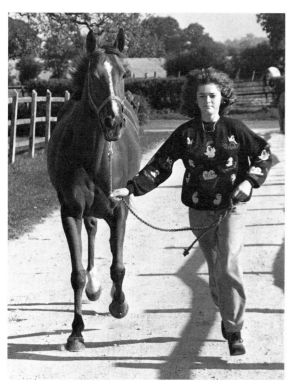

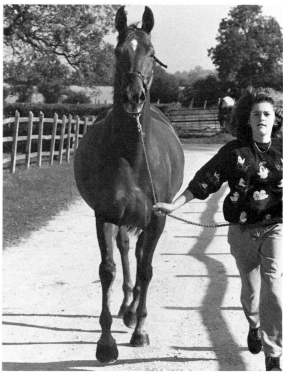

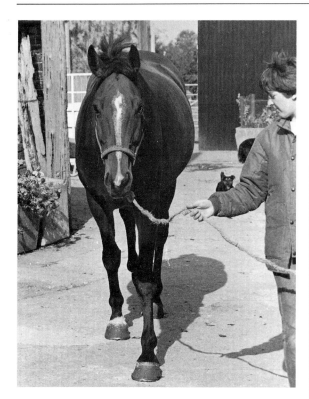

This horse is pigeon-toed, i.e. it turns both feet inwards. It moves very close in front with a crossing action known as 'plaiting'.

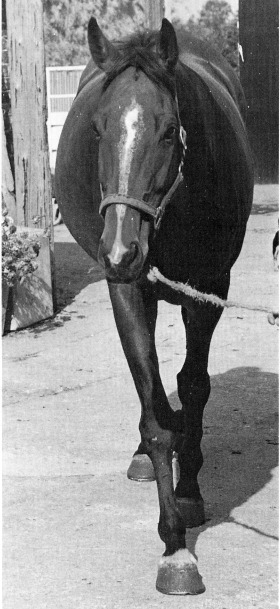

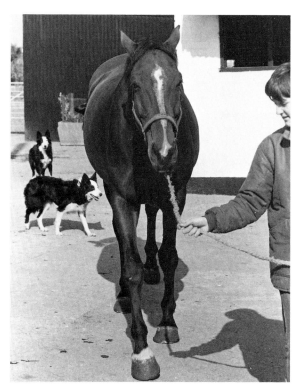

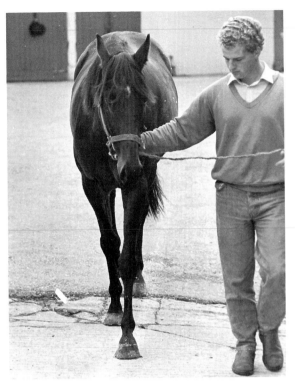

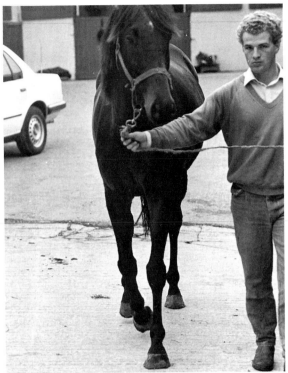

ABOVE: A young horse built so narrow in front that it goes very close, almost to the point of knocking into itself. With maturity and fitness it may improve slightly.

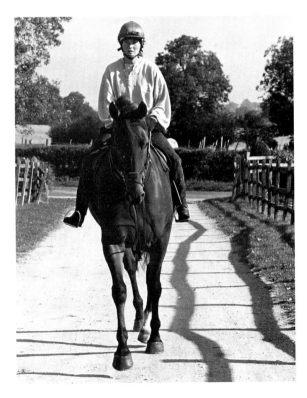

A nice swinging walk. This horse has good chest room but is inclined to cross behind.

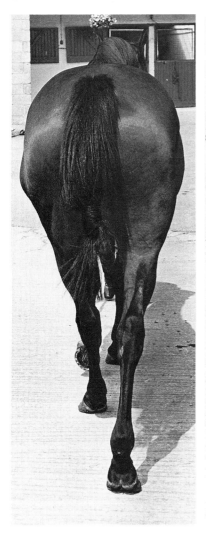

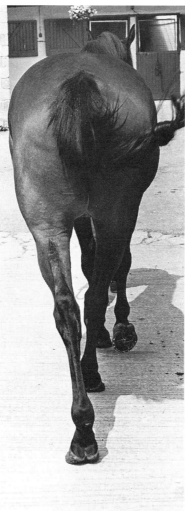

FAR LEFT: Horse moving away. This individual is base narrow, which is surprising from such big, well-muscled hindquarters.

LEFT: The same horse crossing badly behind and dishing in front with the off fore. It would need to wear boots for any competitive work.

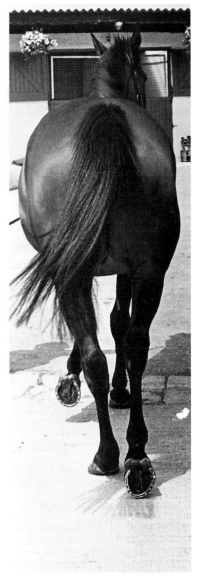

At trot, distinctly showing bad dishing movement in front and about to knock into himself behind.

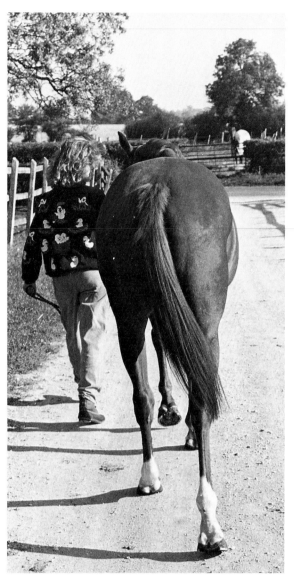
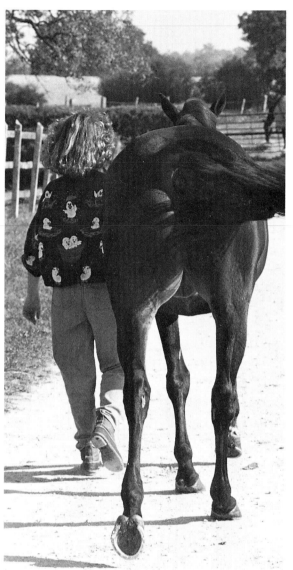

An example of an animal that goes wide behind. Some are born this way, others appear wide behind when over-ridden at the trot causing them to leave their hocks behind. Note the natural swing of the hindquarters and the tail, which is good.

Another example of wide movement behind.

BREEDS AND TYPES

This section features a collection of photographs of horse and pony breeds and types. The purpose is not so much to catalogue the wide variety of individual breeds, but to show how different characteristics and points of conformation come together to create the forms we recognise as breeds or types.

Champion heavyweight hunter – 17 hh, 9 inches of bone, Irish bred.

The animals selected are all typical specimens, and all are major prize winners. Whilst no horse or pony is ever perfect, the animals depicted here are all fine representatives of their breed or type.

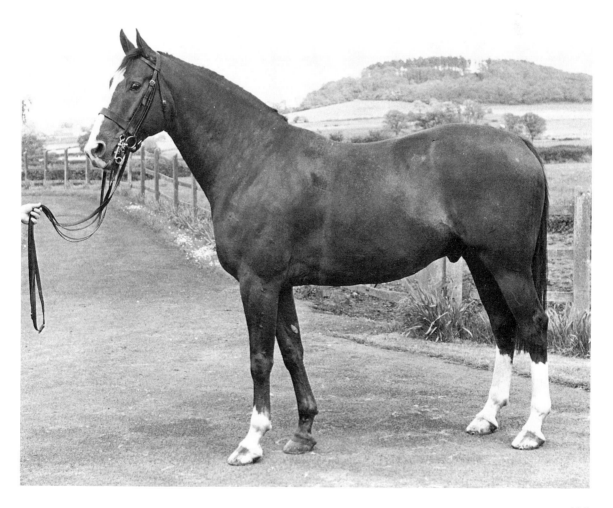

Champion middleweight hunter – 16.3 hh, 8¾ inches of bone, thoroughbred.

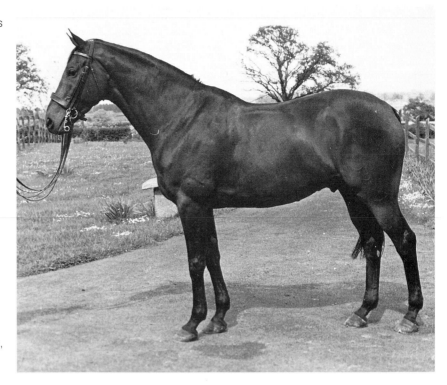

BELOW: Champion lightweight hunter – 16.1 hh, 8½ inches of bone, Irish bred.

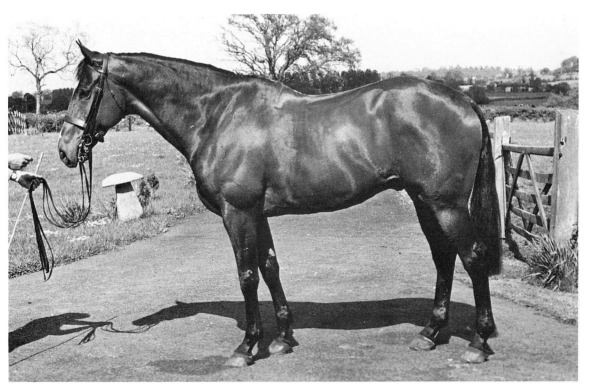

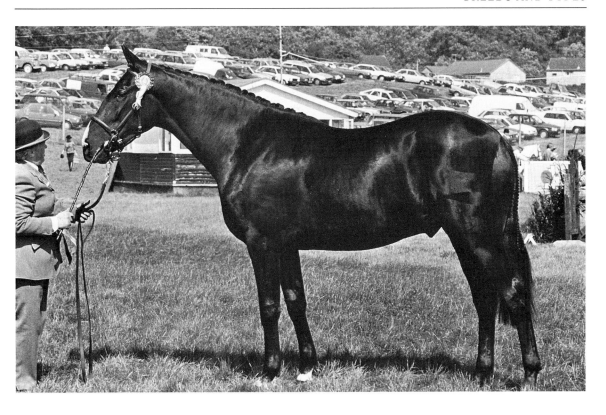

ABOVE: In-hand hunter
champion.

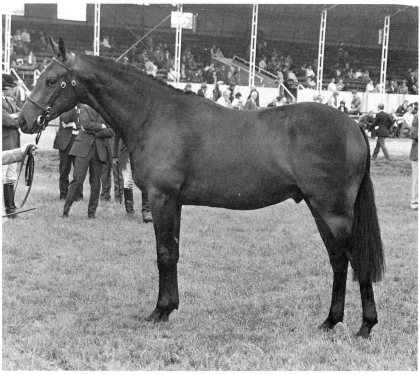

Three-year-old in-hand
hunter champion.

Champion small riding
horse.

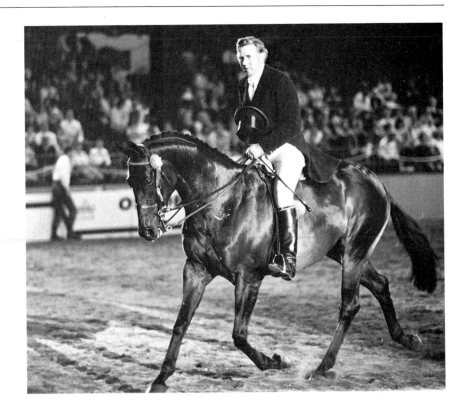

Champion large riding
horse.

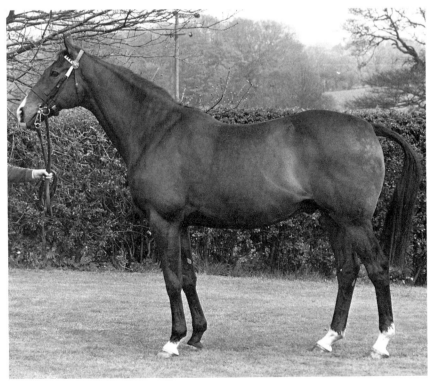

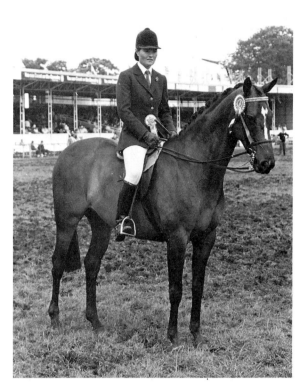

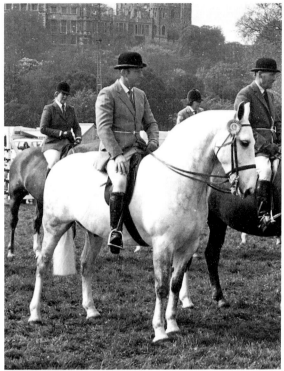

ABOVE: Champion large show hack.

ABOVE, RIGHT: Heavyweight cob champion.

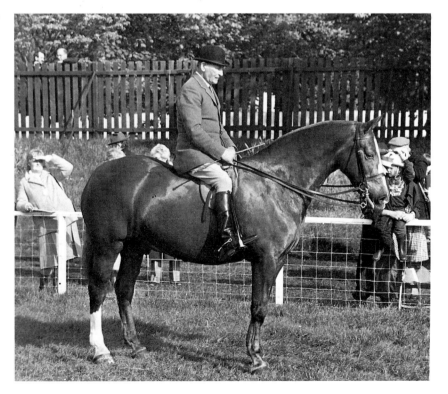

Lightweight cob champion.

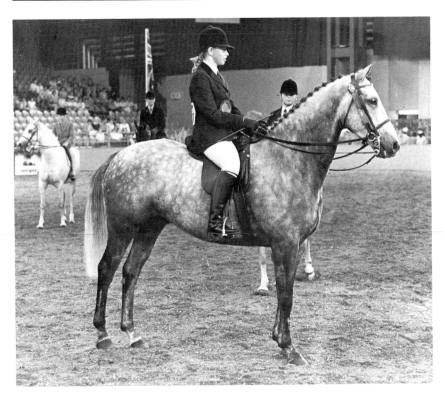

Champion show hunter
pony.

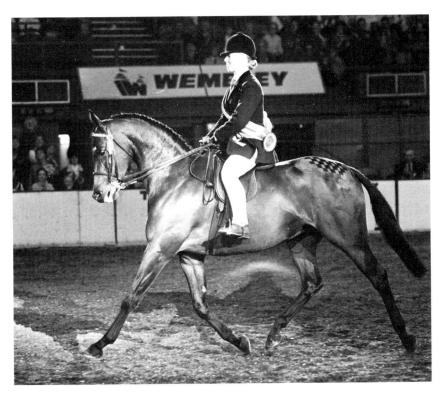

Champion child's ridden
pony.

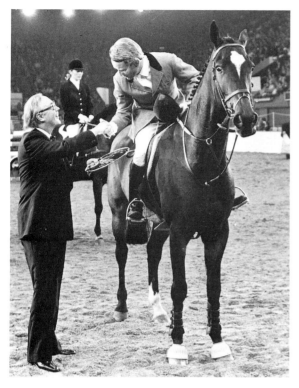

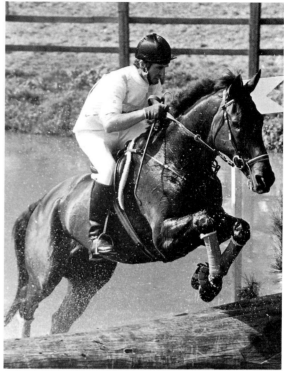

ABOVE: Foxhunter champion.

ABOVE RIGHT: Olympic event horse in action.

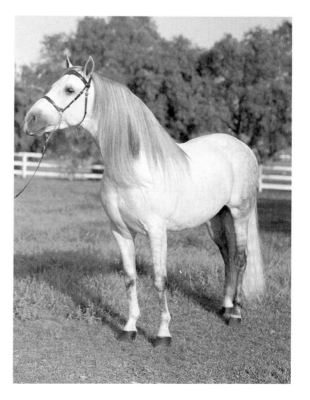

Andalusian stallion.

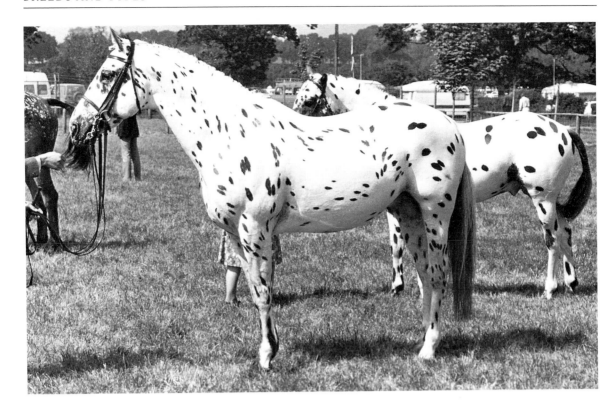

ABOVE: Appaloosa.

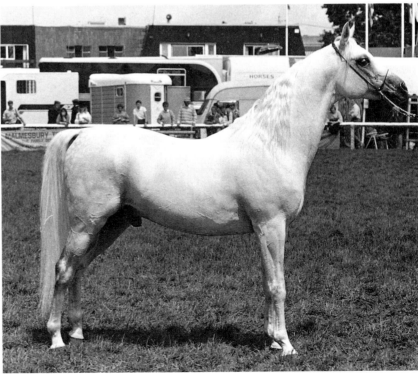

Arab standing up for the judge.

Arab in action in the show ring.

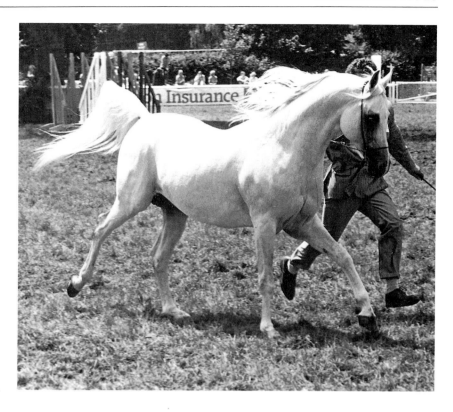

BELOW: Cleveland Bay mare.

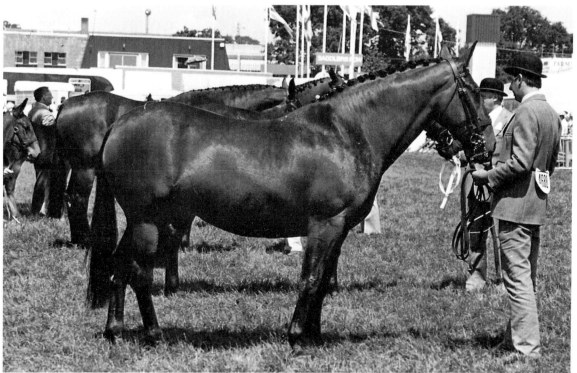

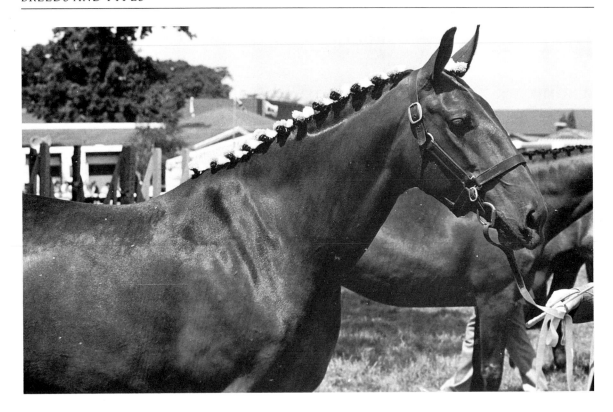

ABOVE: Typical head of a Cleveland Bay.

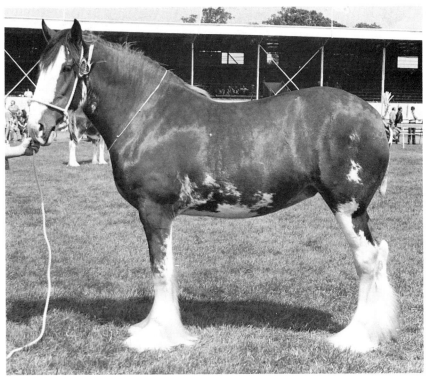

Champion Clydesdale.

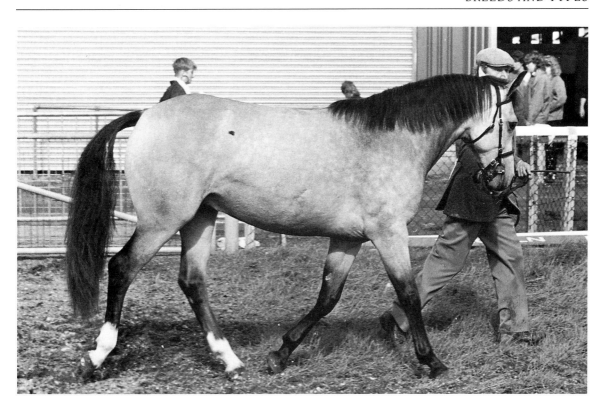

<small>ABOVE:</small> Connemara.

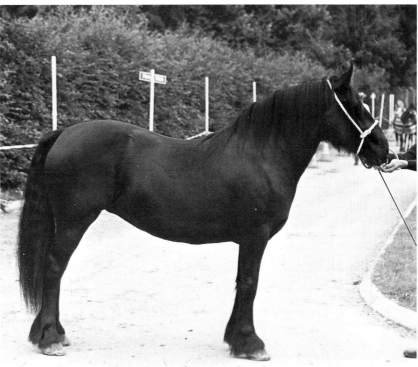

Dales.

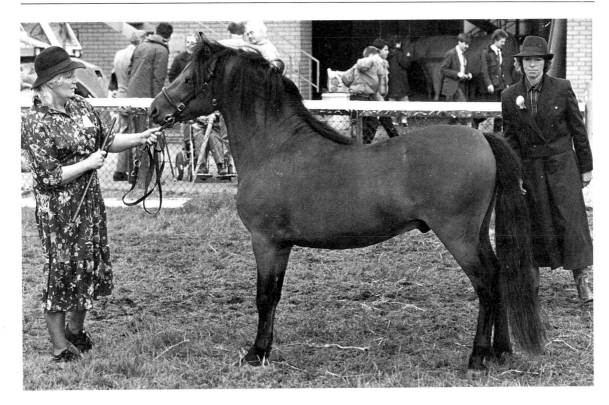

ABOVE: Dartmoor.

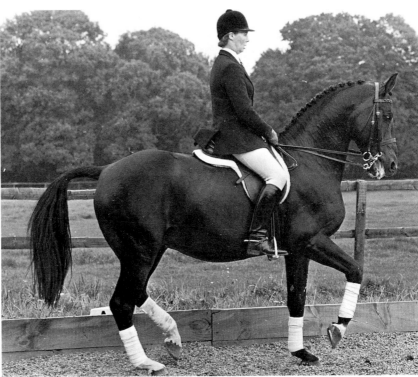

Dutch warmblood stallion.

136

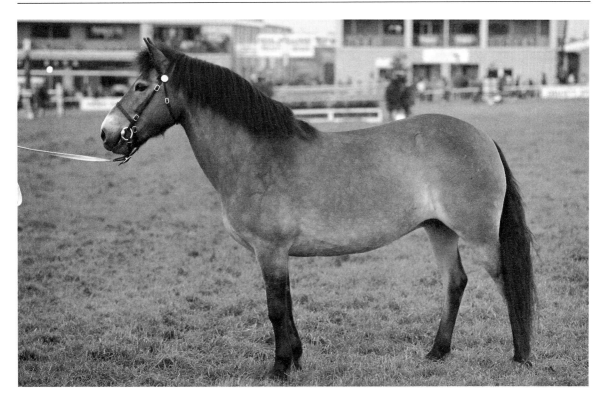

ABOVE: Exmoor champion.

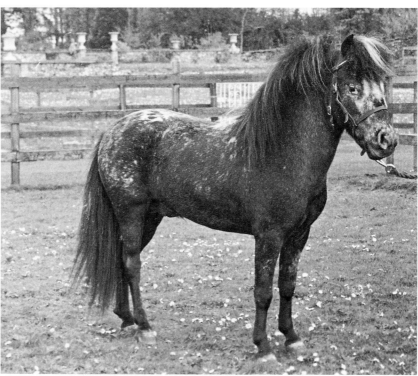

Falabella.

Fell.

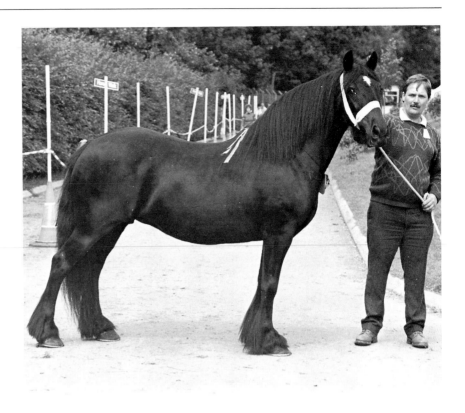

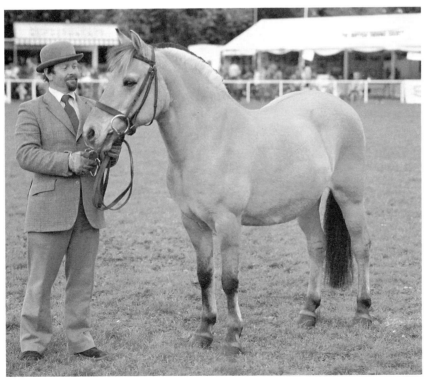

Champion Fjord pony.

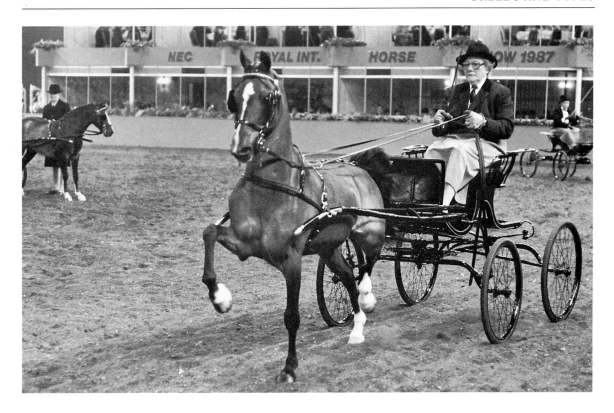

ABOVE: Champion Hackney pony.

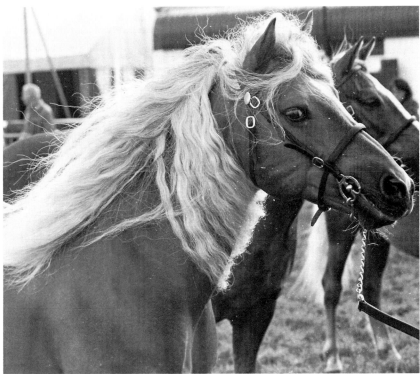

Haflinger.

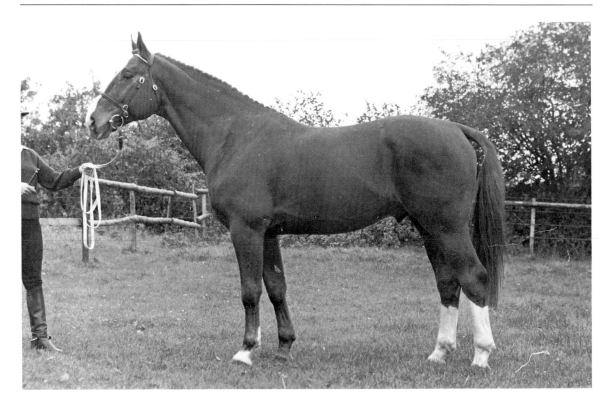

ABOVE: Hanoverian.

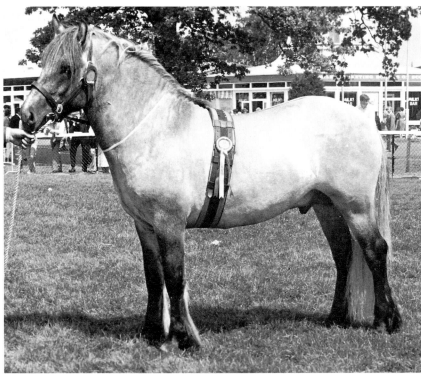

Champion Highland.

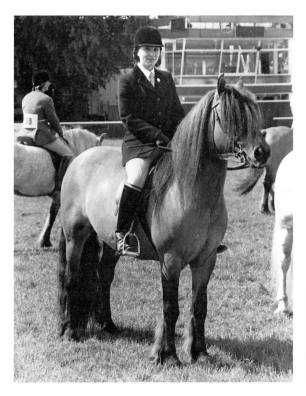

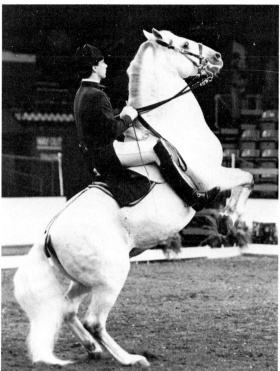

ABOVE: Under 14 hh ridden Highland.

ABOVE, RIGHT: Lipizzaner performing a levade.

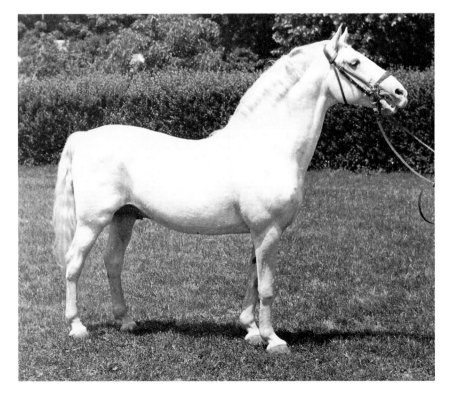

Lipizzaner.

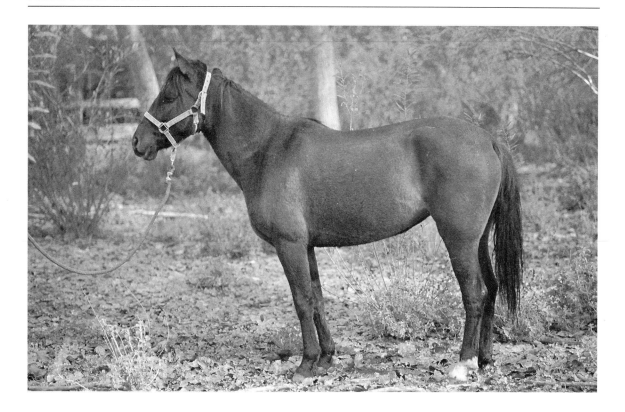

ABOVE: Mustang.

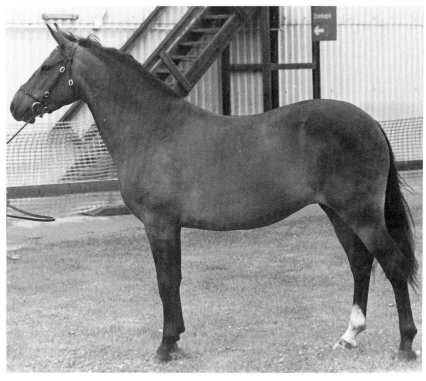

New Forest.

142

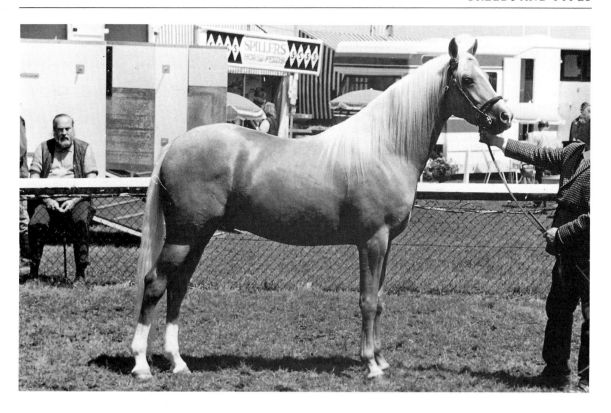

ABOVE: Palomino.

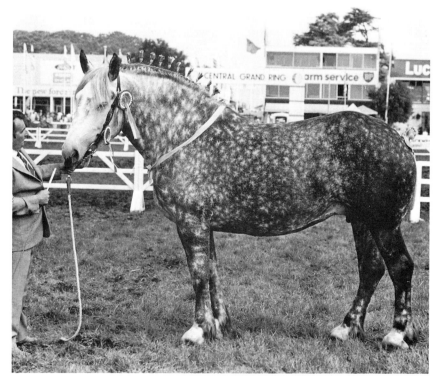

Percheron.

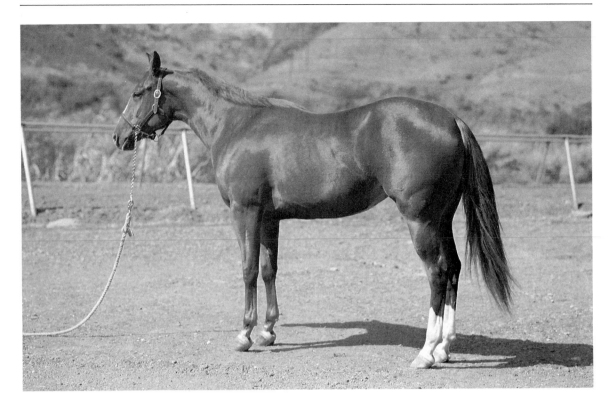

ABOVE: Quarter horse.

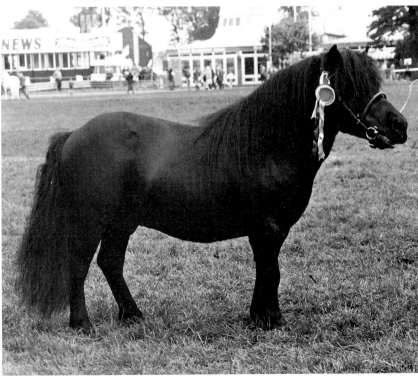

Shetland champion.

Champion Shire.

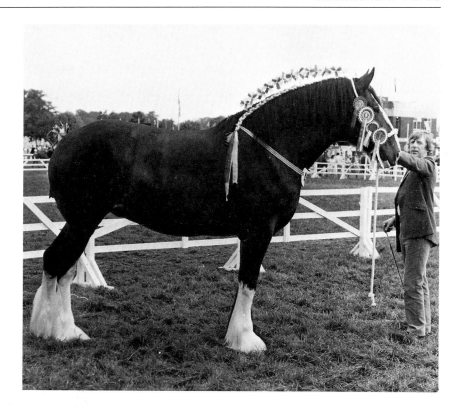

BELOW: Champion Suffolk.

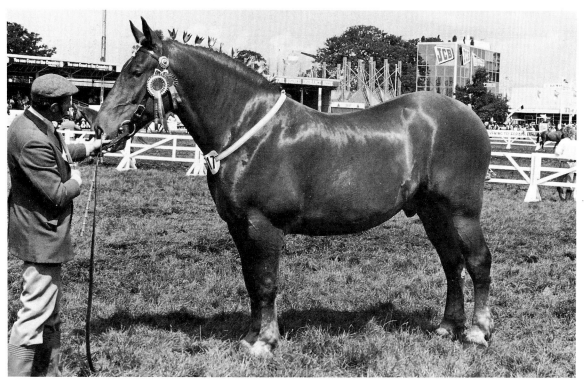

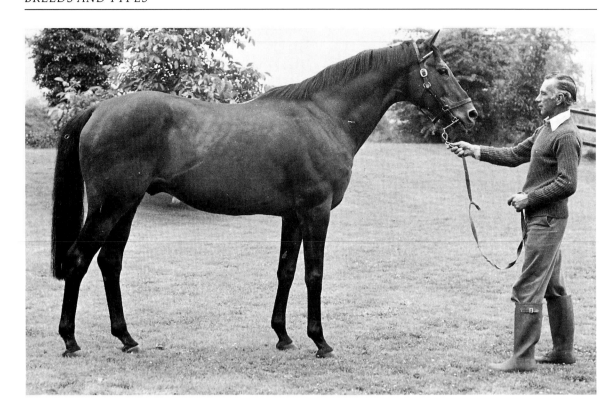

ABOVE: Thoroughbred
stallion.

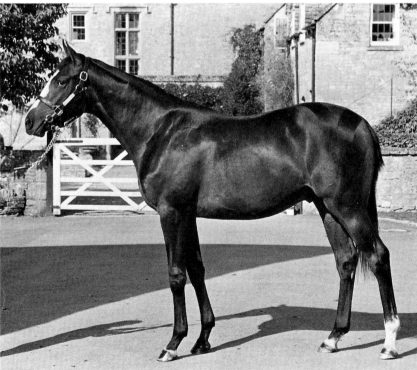

Two-year-old thoroughbred
showing quality and class.

146

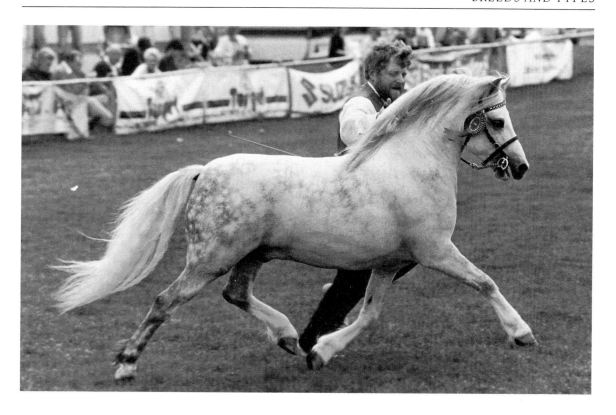

ABOVE: Welsh Section A stallion.

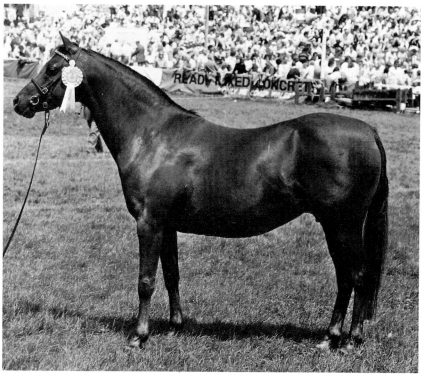

Welsh Section B.

Welsh Section C.

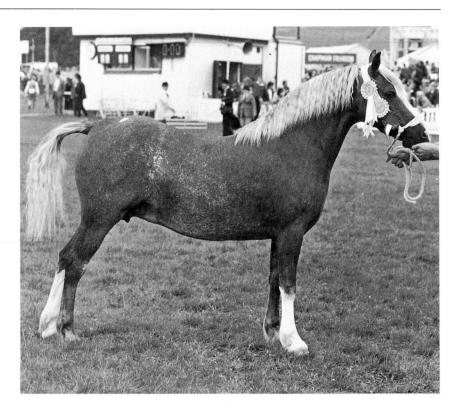

BELOW: Welsh Section D.

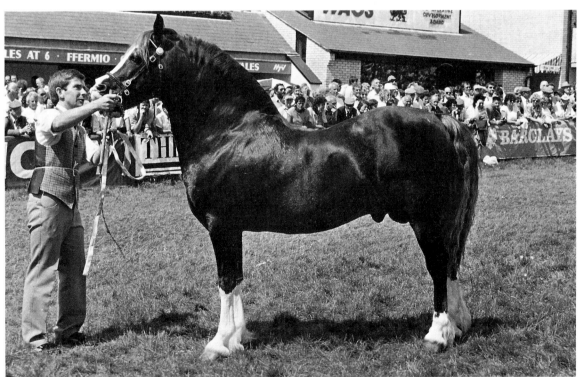

BIBLIOGRAPHY

BURGER, UDO, *The Way to Perfect Horsemanship*, J. A. Allen, London, 1986.

GOODY, PETER C., *Horse Anatomy – A Pictorial Approach to Equine Structure*, J. A. Allen, London, 1983.

HARTLEY EDWARDS, ELWYN, *The Horseman's Manual*, J. A. Allen, London, 1990.

HOLDERNESS-RODDAM, JANE, *Colours and Markings*, Threshold Books, London, 1987.

HUGHES, CHRISTINE and OLIVER, ROBERT, *Practical Stable Management*, Pelham Books, London, 1987.

OLIVER, ROBERT, *Showing Horses and Ponies*, Pelham Books, London, 1985.

RUSSELL, VALERIE, *Judging Horses and Ponies*, Pelham Books, London, 1978.

SMYTHE, R. H., *The Horse: Structure and Movement*, second edition revised by P. C. Goody, J. A. Allen, London, 1975.

SPOONER, GLENDA, *The Handbook of Showing*, revised edition, J. A. Allen, London, 1990.

SUMMERHAYS, R. S., *Summerhays' Encyclopaedia for Horsemen*, revised edition, Threshold Books, London, 1988.

THORNE, JOHN and SUSAN, *Winning with Hunter Ponies*, J. A. Allen, London, 1989.

GLOSSARY

A

Aged   Describes a horse when it reaches the age of seven years or over.

A good doer   A horse that usually looks well on a minimum of food; frequently a pony or cob type.

Albino   A congenital deficiency of colouring pigment in the horse's hair and skin, which results in white hair, pink skin and blue (sometimes brown) eyes. True albinos are rarely seen.

Apple joints   Term used to describe round joints or those which are thick and lumpy. Can be caused by overwork when young but is often an hereditary fault of conformation.

B

Back at the knee/back of the knee   A fault of the forelegs in which the lower limb below the knee (if viewed from the side) tends towards concavity. A limb so built would be of little use in absorbing concussion. Undesirable and unsightly. Also known as 'calf-knee' and 'buck-knee'.

Balance   A horse is said to be balanced when its own weight and that of its rider are distributed over each leg in such a way as to allow the horse to use itself with maximum ease and efficiency in all gaits.

Barrel   The body of the horse, from behind the forearms to the loins.

Base narrow   When viewed from behind or in front, the legs are very close together.

Base wide   When viewed from behind or in front, the horse appears to have a wide space between the legs.

Bishoping   The illegal practice of filing a horse's teeth to give a false impression of the animal's age.

Black points   A term used when describing a horse whose mane, tail, and lower legs are black.

Blemish   Permanent marks or scars appearing on any part of the horse, caused by injury. Most frequently such marks appear on the limbs.

Blue-eye   See WALL-EYE.

Bog spavin   Puffy enlargement at the inner and upper part of the hock joint, caused by strain of the hock. If lame the swelling is hot and painful.

Bone spavin   Bony deposit on the inside and lower part of the hock; may be due to strain. Can be detected by comparing the hocks. Does not always cause lameness but affected horses often drag their hind toes. Lameness decreases with exercise.

Boney hock   A term used when the bone of the hock, when viewed from the side, appears prominent, like a false curb, whereas in fact it does not protrude to form a curb.

Bosomy   When viewed from the side the chest appears abnormally prominent; from the front it looks unusually heavy and wide.

Bone   A horse's 'bone' is measured just below the knee. A lightweight hunter, for example, might have a measurement of 8½ inches.

Bow knees   When viewed from the front, the horse's front legs appear wide just above the knees.

Bowed hocks   When viewed from behind the hocks bow outwards – a weakness.

Boxy feet   Small, donkey-like feet.

Bridle lame Horses so affected appear lame when ridden but sound when trotted up in hand. Caused by over-schooling.

Brisket Lower part of the chest.

Broken knees Injured knees caused by the horse falling or hitting the road and leaving permanent scarring. Causes: long toes through neglect of regular shoeing; slovenly action; stumbling; poor conformation.

Brushing Injury to front or hind inside joints caused when the horse is in motion, and the inner side of the foot strikes the opposite leg. The problem is accentuated by horses that move close.

Buck-knee See BACK AT THE KNEE.

Bull-necked Short and very thick in the neck, seen in common horses, especially cob types.

Butty Descriptive of a short-legged, short-backed, deep-bodied horse. Usually applied to small hunters and cobs.

C

Calf-knee See BACK AT THE KNEE.

Capped elbows Small or large swellings on the elbows, often caused from lying on heels.

Capped hocks Large or small swellings on the point of the hock caused by kicking in the stable or while travelling, or through a shortage of bedding.

Carty Common, cold-blooded draught-horse type.

Cat hairs Long untidy hairs along the line of the jaw, often seen in common horses after clipping.

Churn-barrelled Well ribbed up.

Clean-legged A term applied to quality horses with no hair in their heels or to animals whose legs are blemish-free.

Close-coupled Describes a short-backed, deep-bodied horse.

Club-foot Small, upright foot.

Cock-throttled Describes a horse whose head and neck are badly set on, the line of the gullet convex and similar to that of a cockerel.

Coffin-headed A common, ugly head which lacks a pronounced jowl.

Cold-back Refers to a horse which dislikes a cold saddle placed upon its back. It may react by arching its back to the point of bucking, or by lowering its back to the point of not being able to walk forward. The problem can be alleviated by using a numnah or leaving the saddle loosely girthed for a while before mounting.

Colt Ungelded male horse up to four years old.

Condition State of health and body.

Confidential A horse or pony suitable for a novice or elderly rider.

Conformation A horse's make and shape.

Contracted heels A defect frequently associated with navicular disease. The heels are very narrow and often the frog is not in contact with the ground.

Coronary band A band, or 'cushion', of tissue at the top of the wall of the hoof.

Cow-hocked When viewed from behind hocks appear close together and the hind legs point outwards.

Cresty Having a thick convex neck, as seen in stallions.

Croup Top of hindquarters.

Curb A blemish and an unsoundness, frequently found on bent, badly shaped hocks but also occasionally on the best of hocks. It is an enlargement, varying in size from a pea to an egg, usually found about three or four inches below the point of the hock. Curbs seem to cause less trouble if a horse is born with them than if they arise as a result of a strain.

D

Daisy-cutting Action which is low to the ground with little elevation. Often seen in show ponies.

Dappled Dark spotted markings, often seen on greys.

Dipped back A back that is hollow behind and

in front of the saddle. A weakness but often a good ride.

Dish-faced   Arab-like profile to the head, concave below the eye.

Dishing   Faulty action wherein the foot is thrown outward and forward. It is unsightly when viewed from the front. Horses that dish often have large splints.

Dock   The flesh and bone part of the tail.

Docking   The practice of severing the lower part of the tail; illegal in Britain since 1948.

Donkey-footed   Small, narrow feet together with pinched-in heels.

E

Eel stripe   A dark stripe along the back, often seen in duns.

Elk lip   A heavy, overhanging top lip.

Entire   A male horse which has not been castrated; a stallion.

Ergot   A hard, corn-like growth at the back of the fetlock joint.

Ermine marks   Small black or brown marks on white socks (resembling ermine fur) surrounding the coronet.

Ewe neck   The crest of the neck (i.e. between the poll and the withers) is concave rather than convex; an upside-down neck.

F

False curb   A hock which, when viewed from behind, looks like a curby hock but the 'curb' does not extend to the back of the hock (as a true curb).

'Favouring a leg'   Pointing a front leg forwards, or resting a hind leg.

Feather   Long hair on the lower limbs, especially in the heels. Most frequently seen in heavy horses.

Fiddle-headed   A horse with a large, long, plain head.

Filly   A female horse up to three years old.

Flank   Part of the body behind the ribs.

Flat bone   A term used to describe legs and knees which have a hard, chiselled appearance; the reverse of round bone.

Flat-catcher   A showy, usually fine-coated, good mover whose faults in conformation are belied by its outward good looks. Usually bought by the inexperienced, to the unscrupulous dealer's delight.

Flat-footed   Horses so described have low heels often accompanied by a large foot and large, soft frogs. Difficult to keep sound on stony ground.

Flat-sided   A horse whose ribs are not rounded. Also called slab-sided.

Flea-bitten   A grey coat flecked with hairs of a darker shade.

Flecked   Small collections of white hairs occurring on the body.

Flesh marks   Hairless patches where skin pigment is absent.

Foal   A young horse or pony up to twelve months old.

Footy or fudgy   A term used to describe horses which are not necessarily lame but short striding. They usually go better on a soft surface and improve after warming up.

Forearm   Part of the front leg, from the elbow to the knee.

Forehand   The head, neck, shoulders, withers and forelegs of a horse.

Forging   Collision of the hind shoe with the front shoe when a horse is trotting. Recognised by the clicking noise made as one shoe strikes the other. Often noticed in young or tired horses.

Frog   Soft, V-shaped tissue on the underside of the horse's foot.

Front   The part of the horse in front of the rider when in the saddle.

Fudgy   See FOOTY.

G

Galvayne's groove A brown mark which appears on the corner incisor tooth after the horse is ten years old.

Gaskin Another name for the second thigh which, viewed from behind, can be easily seen as the muscular development outside and above the level of the hocks extending upwards to the buttocks.

Gelding A castrated horse.

Gingering An old trick used by unscrupulous dealers, whereby ginger or some other irritant was placed under a horse's tail to make the horse carry its tail higher.

Girth The circumference of the horse's body behind the withers.

Goose-rumped Describes a horse whose quarters slope acutely from the highest point down to the dock. Also referred to as a 'jumper's bump'.

Grass belly Large swelling of the stomach due to being out at grass or resting.

Green A horse whose education is not complete; a novice.

Grunting An old-fashioned method of testing a horse's wind in the stable. The horse is threatened with a blow from a stick and if unsound will grunt in its fright as it moves away from the impending strike. In former days dealers swore by this method, which is still used today in Ireland.

H

Half-bred A horse which is of unknown breeding or a mixture of breeds; not eligible for entry in the General Stud Book.

Hand The unit of measurement by which the horse's height (taken from the highest point of the wither to the ground) is determined. One hand equals 4 inches.

Heart room Depth through the horse's girth.

Heavy top Describes a coarse neck and shoulders which are out of proportion with the rest of the horse.

Herring-gutted A horse who runs up light and has an exaggerated slope from elbow to stifle, rather like a greyhound; when saddled up girths are prone to slip backwards; deficient of heart and lung room and therefore seldom a good stayer out hunting.

HH Hands high. See also HAND.

High blowing A distinctive sound sometimes heard when a horse is galloping. It is caused by the flapping of the alae of the nostrils. Can be mistaken for roaring (q.v.) by inexperienced horsemen but has no connection with the disease and can be disregarded.

Hip down When viewed from behind, one hip appears to have dropped lower than the other; wasted muscle is noticed on the lower side.

Hips, ragged The points of the horse's hips are very prominent.

Hobdayed Describes a horse which has been operated on to relieve roaring or whistling.

Hollow-backed Describes a back which dips behind the withers. A conformation fault which usually gives a comfortable ride. Can be due to age and hard work but is also found in young horses.

Hock The joint between the second thigh and the hind cannon.

Hocks, cow Hocks which are set very close together when viewed from behind. Also, feet turn out.

Hocks, curby Bent, badly shaped hocks prone to curbs, or those with a curb actually present.

Hocks, sickle Bent and weak hocks.

Hocks, sprung Hocks which are puffy and swollen from accident or wear.

Hocks, well-let-down The hocks look close to the fetlock joints.

Hocks in the air The opposite of well-let-down hocks, with long cannon bones.

Hocks in the next county Hocks are set way out behind the horse's body. Unsightly.

Hog back See ROACH BACK.

Hogged mane A mane which has been completely shorn off.

Hoof Horse's foot covered in horny grown from coronet downwards.

Horn Outer surface of the foot; also called the wall of the foot.

I

Incisors The front, biting teeth. The horse's age can be assessed from their appearance.

Interfering Faulty action when one foot knocks the joint of another.

J

Jowl The upper part of the horse's jaw.

Jumper's bump See GOOSE-RUMPED.

K

Knee The joint between the forearm and the cannon bone.

Knocking Same as BRUSHING (q.v.)

L

Lacing Same as PLAITING (q.v.).

Legs, filled Swollen or puffy legs caused from over-work or over-feeding.

Legs, gammy/gummy As LEGS, FILLED (above); usually the result of incorrect feeding.

Legs out of one hole A description of a horse that is narrow-chested and goes close in front.

Let down Describes a well-conditioned horse, the opposite of one that looks tucked up.

Light of bone The bone below the knee is small in proportion to the size of the horse.

Limbs Horseman's term for the lower half of the leg.

List A dark stripe along the back.

Loaded shoulder Excessive thickness over the shoulders (wide and heavy).

Loins On the horse's back, the space immediately behind the saddle.

'Long in the tooth' Describes an old horse, whose front teeth have literally grown long.

Lop ears Ears that are floppy, placed wide apart and dropping downwards. Considered ugly but often found on genuine horses.

M

'Makes a noise' Unsound in wind. See also ROARER and WHISTLING.

Mark Refers to the dark centre of a young horse's tooth.

Mealy Oatmeal colouring found especially on the muzzles of Exmoor ponies.

Mouldy A mouldy sort of horse is one that is a very good model, round and attractive.

Muzzle Part of the head, which includes the nose and mouth.

Mule feet Small, boxy feet.

N

Nappy A horse which refuses to go forwards through bad temper or stubbornness, e.g. declines to leave its stable or the company of other horses.

Narrow behind Hind legs set very close together.

Narrow in front Front legs set very close together with no chest room.

Near side The left-hand side of the horse; the right-hand side is called the off side.

'No foot, no horse' An old horseman's expression and the best advice anyone can have. However good an animal may appear, if its feet are not good, trouble is bound to follow.

Nostril Part of the nose, through which the horse breathes.

Novice   In showing, a horse that has not won a first prize of a certain value; otherwise, a horse that has not won a competition.

Nut-cracker   A horse that has the habit of grinding its teeth, usually when under pressure from a rider whilst being schooled.

O

Off side   The right-hand side of the horse; the left-hand side is called the near side.

On the leg   A phrase describing a tall horse whose body seems to be carried on stilts, so that it shows too much daylight underneath.

Open knees   Knees which have a horizontal groove through their centre, often apparent in young racehorses.

Out at elbow   A horse whose elbows project outwards.

Over at the knee   A forward bend or curve of the knee; can be a conformation fault or caused by excessive wear.

Overshot mouth   See PARROT MOUTH.

Over-topped   Describes a horse whose body appears large and out of proportion to its body. Often associated with horses that are light of bone. The problem is accentuated when a horse is carrying too much weight.

P

'Past mark of mouth'   An expression denoting an aged horse.

Pasterns   Part of the horse's leg between the fetlock joint and the hoof. Should be neither too short nor too long.

'Patent safety'   A quiet, safe, reliable horse or pony.

Parrot mouth   Malformation of the upper jaw whereby the front teeth overhang the lower ones. If severe can prevent a horse from grazing or eating normally. Also known as 'overshot'.

Peacocky   A showy horse with a high head carriage. Not favoured by true horsemen.

Pear-shaped   An old-fashioned grooms' term to describe good hindquarters viewed from the rear.

Prophet's thumb mark   An indentation or dimple on the horse's neck, the size of a thumb.

Piebald   A coat which is black and white in patches.

Pig eye   Small, narrow eye.

Pig mouth   The opposite of parrot mouth (q.v.).

Pigeon-toed   See PIN-TOED.

Pin-toed   Toes which turn inwards. Horses with this fault never strike into themselves, whereas horses whose feet turn outwards frequently strike their fetlock joints. Also known as 'pigeon-toed'.

Plaiting   Front or hind feet cross over when in action. A bad fault.

Pointing   The act of pointing a front foot forward while at rest. Can indicate foot trouble, particularly navicular.

Poll   The top of the horse's head, between the ears.

Poverty lines   Well-defined lines from the dock to the second thigh seen in horses in poor condition.

Presence   A quality which few horses possess, but those who have it stand out. It is an essential attribute in a show horse and is often seen in top competition horses—Arkle and Desert Orchid, for example.

Proppy   Moving with a stilted action, possibly due to being straight-shouldered.

Q

Quarters   The body area from flank to top of the tail.

Quarters, drooping   Quarters which slope away behind the croup.

R

Razor-backed   Having a pronounced and sharp back bone.

Ribby Short of condition, the ribs being clearly visible; poor.

Rig A horse with a retained testicle.

Ring bone Bony formation on the lower pastern bones. If it occurs around the pastern joint it is known as 'high ring bone'.

Rising A term used in connection with the age of a horse. A horse said to be nearly three years old would be described as 'rising three'. Often used at the beginning and end of the year.

Roach back A malformed, convex spinal column; also known as 'hog back'.

Roarer A horse that makes a noise when galloping, due to a serious weakness of the larynx. Not to be confused with whistling (q.v.), which is a modified form.

Roman nose A nose which is plain and convex in shape.

S

Scopey A horse that stands over a lot of ground.

Second thigh Also known as gaskin; part of the hind leg between the stifle and the hock. Should be well defined.

Shannon Cannon bone of hind leg.

Shin Front of cannon bone.

Shiverer A term describing a horse which suffers from 'shivering', a disease of the nervous system which affects both hindquarters and regarded as an unsoundness.

'Short of a rib' Long backed.

'Short of bone' Light of bone below the knee.

Short-coupled A term used for short-backed horses, a type favoured by horsemen.

Shoulders See SLOPING SHOULDERS, LOADED SHOULDERS and UPRIGHT SHOULDERS.

Showing daylight Tall, leggy horse.

Showing wear Joints puffy, round and filled.

Sickle hocks Bent and weak-looking hocks which resemble a sickle. A sign of weakness.

Side bone Ossification affecting the pastern. The wings of the bone of the foot feel hard and immoveable; the horse goes on its toes with a shuffling action.

Skewbald A non-uniform coat of brown (generally) and white patches.

Slab-sided See FLAT-SIDED.

Slack loins Weak behind the saddle; 'light' through.

Slipped (or locked) stifle A dislocation of the stifle, which can occur in young or out of condition horses. The leg appears locked behind and cannot be brought forward. Can be improved surgically.

Sloping shoulders A desirable feature since they have an important bearing on the action of the horse and the comfort of the rider.

Snip A white mark on the nose.

Sock White markings on the fetlock joint.

Sole The underside of the horse's foot.

Sore shins Inflammation of the front of the cannon bone; a common cause of lameness among young racehorses. Horses affected appear to be short in action, especially on hard ground.

Sorrel Chestnut coat colour; a US term; also an old-fashioned English term.

Splint Bony growth between the splint bone and cannon bone in either fore or hind limb.

Spavin See BONE SPAVIN and BOG SPAVIN.

Split up behind Describes the rear view of a horse whose hind legs are widely divided.

Stag-eared Describes ears that are set close together; said to indicate a cunning nature.

Star Small white mark on the forehead.

Star gazer A horse that carries its head unnaturally high; frightening to ride over large fences.

Staring coat A sign of illness: the coat stands on end and loses its lustre.

Stifle Joint between tibia and patella.

Stocking White marking extending down the cannon bones to the foot.

Stringhalt Nervous affliction of the hock, causing one or both hind legs to be lifted in a high, jerking action. Can make horses difficult to shoe and to rein-back. The problem is incurable and gets worse with age.

Stripe Narrow white marking running down the face.

Stripe, dorsal Dark stripe running along the backbone. Also known as 'eel stripe' or 'list'.

Sway-backed A back that is dipped behind the withers.

T

Tendon Fibrous tissue attaching a muscle to a bone. The horse's tendons should be hard and sinewy, not soft or puffy.

Thick in the wind Describes a horse whose respiration is not as clear as it should be. Horses may become thick in the wind as the result of a cold or unfitness, and their faulty breathing will be more audible when ridden.

Tied in below the knee A bad fault where the measurement immediately below the knee is less than the measurement taken lower down towards the fetlock.

Tied in at the elbow Elbows very close to the ribs.

Thoroughpin A fluid distension above and on either side of the hock.

Top line The profile of the horse's body.

'Touched in the wind' Makes a noise when galloped.

Tubed Describes a horse which has been operated on for its wind (a small hole is made in the windpipe).

Tucked up Light through the middle after hard work.

Tushes Small pointed teeth found just behind the corner incisors; not found in mares. Tushes usually appear from four years old.

U

Undershot jaw The horse's lower jaw projects beyond the upper jaw, creating a faulty bite.

Upright shoulders An undesirable feature since they produce neither good action nor a comfortable ride. They are usually associated with straight, upright pasterns and cause excessive jarring and wear.

'Up to weight' A horse with a lot of bone, capable of carrying a heavy rider.

V

Vanner A common-bred animal used in the past as a milk and bread delivery horse. Cobby in type and about 15–15.2 hh.

Varminty An attractive, cheeky-looking horse.

W

Wall eye Lack of pigment in the iris, giving a pinkish-white or bluish-white appearance to the eye. Not an indication of blindness.

Weed A long-legged animal, unimpressive in appearance with poor, mean conformation. Usually a thoroughbred type with very little bone.

Well let down The horse's body is close to the ground (i.e. with short legs). Also used to describe a horse that is in good condition.

Well ribbed up An expression used to describe a horse that is well rounded with a minimum of space between the last rib and the hip.

Whistling An unsoundness which causes the horse's vocal chords to vibrate in the air stream of the larynx, emitting a distinctive noise. See also ROARER.

White-faced The whole of the front of the face is white.

Whole-coloured Devoid of white markings; all of one colour.

Whorl Small areas of irregular coat growth, most frequently found on the head, neck and chest of the horse; they are useful aids in identification.

Wide behind Describes the rear view of an animal whose hind legs, from the feet upwards, are set wide apart. Also describes movement behind which is wide.

Windgalls Soft, round painless swellings above and behind the fetlock joint on both sides of the limb. Caused by wear and tear, they are unsightly but of no consequence.

Withers These commence at the base of the neck and slope away into the back.

Wobbler Foal born unable to stand properly; youngstock so afflicted rarely survive.

Wolf teeth Rudimentary teeth which can appear in front of the upper molars. They serve no useful purpose and are best removed.

Y

Yawd North Country term for an ugly, useless type of horse usually of unknown breeding.

Yawing Describes the action of a horse who when ridden fights with its head to reach outwards and downwards.

Z

Zebra marks Stripes on the legs, neck and withers. Rare.

INDEX